PATIENT
TEACHERS

John W. Burnside, M.D.

ISBN: 1500490873
ISBN 13: 9781500490874

This book is dedicated to all the patients who have taught me so much about the human condition and allowed a crowd of medical students and residents to invade their space and hear the most intimate details of their lives.

PREFACE

These stories have been written over the course of 45 years of medical practice. They begin during my internship and residency at the Massachusetts General Hospital in Boston from 1966 through 1971. They are designated "Boston" under the title. The next series are from The Pennsylvania State University College of Medicine from 1971 through 1989 and are designated "Hershey". The last are from 1989 through 2000 at the University of Texas Southwestern Medical School in Dallas and are designated "Dallas" The final designation of "Miscellany" are musings throughout and are not about specific patients.

I have been blessed to witness extraordinary changes in the understanding of diseases, the application of great new technologies, techniques and pharmacies. You will recognize some relatively primitive efforts in the early stories. What have not changed are the elements of the human condition.

TABLE OF CONTENTS

IRA AND THE GYPSY

BOSTON

I ra got the Gypsy. Ira measured five feet five inches. So did the Gypsy. Ira weighed 130 pounds. The Gypsy did not. She would have been kindly served by weight measured in stones - the number would have been less intimidating. As it was, she was too heavy to weigh on a conventional scale and too sick to take to the loading dock for the commercial scale.

Ira Bronstein and I were resident physicians together. We worked together alternating admissions every other day and night for two years. This mutual immersion was occasioned by nothing more that the proximity of our surnames on the alphabetical list. Educational partnerships are always like this. Four at a lab bench would have the same first letter and so it was with the call schedule for resident training. A try to match dispositions or interests would be futile so it's as good a system as any. You learn a great deal about your comrade and yourself when you spend time in the marathon dance called residency training.

Ira was not only wispy in size he was very young. Accelerated training for the gifted allowed Ira to complete college and medical school in six years. I learned why the usual curriculum takes eight years from my association with Ira. The sages of yesteryear who so decreed probably felt that doctors, at least male doctors, would inspire more confidence in their patients if their voice had fully changed. Ira's voice broke with regularity. He suffered in other ways too. He could never garner the sympathy of his attending physicians by showing up for morning rounds with noticeable stubble on his chin - the badge that said, "Hey guys, I worked so hard last night, I couldn't even shave this morning".

In fact, Ira never looked tired. He brimmed with energy - a kind of static charge, not terribly focused just crackling at the touch. His gait emphasized his stature and his energy. He overstepped and bounded up on the balls of his feet as if in prelaunch. I suspect he selected internal medicine because it was more cerebral than surgery and besides his clumsiness would be less an impediment.

Ira was a genius but he wasn't very smart. Convinced that the entire human condition could be reduced to manageable mathematical terms, Ira attacked clinical medicine with a slide rule (this was circa 1967 - it would have been wonderful to watch him with pocket calculator and computer). Ira doodled with differential equations. If he lusted it was not for that succulent nurse on the third floor who favored all interns with an occasional "Oops, scuse me" brush of soft breast against the arm. It would have been the Ira Bronstein Unifying Theory of Life and Death - with footnotes - that would make him breathe hard.

The large Gypsy beached in the emergency room on a warm summer evening. I was tending to a patient with a gastro-intestinal bleed and became aware of a substantial commotion in the next cubicle separated by a draw curtain. There was a combination of bleating cries and grunts and a flapping of the curtain. I pulled the curtain back a bit and looked in. The Gypsy was a corpulent mass draped somewhat precariously on a relatively thin stretcher. Her jiggling panniculus threatened to spill over the side and siphon her to the floor like some giant slinky. Surrounding her were swarthy men, tiny dark haired women and a few doe eyed children. I could just see Ira squeezing through this forest of bodies with panic in his eyes. I pulled him aside and we went into the resident's room to get it together.

"Got a big one there Ira", I said hoping to quiet him with nonchalance.

"She's a Queen!" gasped Ira. "A Gypsy Queen. They'll probably kill me if I screw up."

"No Ira. You'll be famous when you get her well", I said. I had been here before and Ira had not. Every Gypsy who gets admitted to the hospital is a queen if a woman or king if a man. Perhaps that's what decides who shall reign. More likely these master survivors have learned that such a designation garners a bit more attention. It clearly had Ira's attention. "Get the room cleared of all those people and finish your examination. Then let's talk."

An hour or so later, I found Ira back in the resident's room. He seemed more in control and was making notations and sliding his rule.

"Everything OK Ira?"

"Uh, yes. She's in congestive heart failure - probably hypertensive heart disease - maybe some renal failure - have to wait for the labs - want to get her up to the floor", he stuttered in staccato. "Found a vein - got an I.V. started - gave her some diuretics." His head bobbed with increasing enthusiasm for the task. He went on to give me his calculations for her total body sodium stores, body surface area and displacement, drug distribution curves for his ordered drugs and a few more calculations to salve his uncertainty.

"Got a Foley catheter in her bladder to measure her urine output?" I asked mischievously, anticipating the response I got.

"Uh, no. Thought I'd wait till we got her upstairs."

The operative condition was that Foley catheters placed in the emergency room were the responsibility of the resident but on the floor they were handled by the nursing staff.

I guess fatigue perverted my sense of humor but I couldn't help chuckling at the visual imagery of Ira trying to place a Foley catheter in the queen. Parked on a stool between gargantuan thighs kneading rolls of flesh and probing for a small urethral meatus. Should her foot slip from the stirrup, Ira would be lost forever.

I forgot about Ira and the Gypsy in the press of another admission, late night rounds, phone calls and a final prayer for a quiet night. That was not to be.

"Code Blue - Bulfinch Three!" I made a sockless dash across the courtyard from the resident's quarters to find the second verse of the emergency room scene. This time a full orchestra with descants, toccatas and fugues. The Gypsy's room was jammed with squirming wailing bodies. I could see Ira perched on the Gypsy's chest. He was astride the queen knees tucked under her lolling breasts. His tiny hands were fisted on her sternum trying to compress both her heart and the intervening suit. Periodically, his head dove forward to give a sticky kiss and blow, successful only in pushing a few pink bubbles from her nose. The bed was lurching not so much from Ira's efforts as from the tugging of the family as they jerked it sideways toward the window across the room.

"Stars! Stars!" I heard it clearly through the din and I knew why. Death under the stars was another of the stage directions from the ages. The Gypsies knew that the queen was dying - was dead. By now the bed was close, Ira dislodged from his perch and the queen was sideways on the bed with the family alternately pulling and pushing till her head was on the sill perched against the glass. The wailing rose in unison and collapsed to a sigh. Everyone departed in groups of two or three now talking quietly with one another like parishioners departing church. A sudden astonishing "Well, that's that. What's for dinner?"

Ira was a mess. He was lost in his oversized OR greens in which we all slept. There were smears of blood and various body fluids all over him, his eyes showed white clear around and his jaw was working up and down soundlessly. Ira was on the fine line.

"Let's get some tea, Ira", I said, remembering that Ira didn't drink the foul thick coffee of the intensive care unit. Slowly, Ira came around. I believe his first intelligible utterance was a query about potassium flux and myocardial contractility and did I think it was significant with the queen.

We talked quietly until fatigue returned and walked together for a last sweep through the intensive care unit. Stopping in the queen's room we found the deiner preparing the body for removal. Ira picked up his white coat and began searching for his slide rule, which was dislodged during the commotion. His distress returned as he searched in vain. I looked about too. Yes the phone headset was gone, the leads to the EKG machine were gone and for final confirmation I looked in the bathroom to note the absence of both rolls of toilet paper. Poor Ira.

GINGSENG MAN

HERSHEY

He was somewhere in his seventies when I first met him. His age was often a question of mine but of no concern of his. That first visit to the office started a 6-year sparring match in which we both took pleasure.

"Good afternoon, Mr. Clemens, my name is Dr. Burnside."
"Otis," he said.
"Beg your pardon?"
"Most folks just call me Otis," he replied.

He was short, solid and smelled musty. He had gray crew-cut hair, and there were defiant tufts from his ears and nostrils. He wore khaki slacks, well-worn high-topped shoes, checked flannel shirt, and a string tie with an Indian clasp. His "dress up tie" I was later to learn.

"What's the problem?" I inquired.
"For you to find out, innit?" he said, looking at me sideways.

Terrific! Six more patients to see, I'm already behind, and this crusty devil wants to play games. Not a very empathetic response but there it was. A labored drill of "yeps" and "nopes" led to the diagnosis of diabetes as his major problem. I took a long time to get there so that I could hardly pursue much else. My exam was abbreviated but enough to confirm the absence of any significant retinopathy or neuropathy, a grade one aortic stenosis murmur, moderately enlarged prostate, and one absent foot pulse. Not too shabby for seventy plus and carbohydrate intolerance.

I told him of some lab tests that I wanted, talked a bit about diabetes, arranged for him to see the dietitian, and set up another appointment. As he was leaving, hand on the door, he turned and with a shy grin said, "You're better'n the last. I may be back."

Over the next 2 weeks, I found Otis popping into my mind at odd moments. I had missed something - no, I had missed a lot. I hoped that he would keep the next appointment. I wondered if I really had passed his secret test. He came.

Over time, he gave me little glimpses of who he was. I was never quite sure if he was teasing me or was just afraid to reveal too much too soon. I discovered a man who had little patience with civilization. Not angry, just self-sufficient and happy to be alone.

> "...live in a cabin on Blue mountain. Built it myself."
> "...wife died a long time ago."
> "...gotta son. Lives in Texas. Writes once in a while."
> "...gotta dog. Good dog."
> "...Hoffer's a good read."
> "...naw, pay ya cash.
> Don't have Medicare, don't draw security."

I found myself responding in kind, telling him little bits about myself. Our conversations were less and less questions and answers and more and more simple declaratives. He was comfortable with silence and taught me to be the same. He would remember these little confidences and bring me things. Once a small meteorite for my sons, a couple of small mountain laurel for my garden, a good book.

We began to have fun, but his diabetes was no better.
Time and again his blood sugars pushed 300. I was certain he was getting up every couple of hours at night to go to his one-holer.

> "Can't piss off the porch. Draws the porcupines. They like the sweet salt."

Talking diet was talking nonsense. He ate when he felt like it and what he felt like - game, fruit, or whatever took his fancy during his infrequent trips to the grocery store. We started oral hypoglycemics - pushed to a maximum dose and still no real response. I really did not like the idea of going to insulin. One episode of low blood sugar on the mountain and that would be the end of Otis.

Coming into the hospital for regulation was hard to contemplate as well. For Otis, personal control was everything and he would not tolerate much tinkering.

Then things started happening. His sugar began to come down to, if not normal levels, acceptable limits.

"Terrific, Otis. Guess that last medication is finally working," I said.

"Nope. Threw the pills away. Just taking Ginseng."

"Ginseng? Otis, you're pulling my leg," I laughed.

He was not. This was his last secret. Ginseng is a small plant long revered in China and Korea for its medicinal qualities. Good as a tonic, for impotence, colds, aches, and pains so the story goes. He told me that ginseng had also been found in the Pennsylvania Appalachian Mountains. In fact, he made his livelihood from this plant. The root is the prized part and must look "human."

He brought me a prime specimen; and indeed there was a central root like a carrot with side roots resembling twisted arms and legs. Circular ridges around the root showed the age of the plant - this one had 30 rings. Otis knew the locations of plants. He would tend them, remember them, and, when they were ready, harvest and dry the roots.

Some went to New York, others to local pow-wow doctors, Oriental food stores and individual customers. A fine root would bring as much as $100.

Otis had recognized the commercial value but was not himself a devotee until he began to use it for his diabetes. He made teas, put powder on his cereal, and would just gnaw on root chips - his sugar came down.

Ridiculous! Not cause and effect, just true - true and unrelated, I was certain. Whatever, I was pleased with the circumstances. Now I found myself a bit like Otis. Shyly and indirectly, I would bring up the topic with my colleagues.

"Ever heard of ginseng? Some guy I know claims ginseng's good for diabetes. What do you think of that?" I said laughingly but secretly looking for a reaction

Otis is dead now. He had a couple of transient ischemic attacks and then succumbed quickly to a myocardial infarction. It was, as the Greeks would have said, a good death. Some time later in the library, I chanced on a journal, Chinese Medicine, devoted to the medicinal properties of ginseng. One learned article showed carefully the blood sugar lowering effects of the herb.

Thanks, Otis

QUERNEVACA

DALLAS

I tell students what my teachers told me. I tell them that the best medicine comes from knowing your patients. Diagnoses are likely to be more accurate when the signs and symptoms can be interpreted in the context of the patient's family and past experiences and when they are filtered through your own screen of understanding of that patient. Complaints of pain in the kvetch mean less than pain in the stoic for instance. I also use this argument in support of primary care or in my case general internal medicine. Selfishly, knowing patients gives me more pleasure than a constant string of new patients seen once or twice then not again.

Once in a while, not knowing is best as Lillian and Andy Gardner taught me. I was asked to see Lillian by a prominent Dallas businessman who knew them both for many years. Lillian, he said, was sick. He didn't know what was wrong and no I couldn't speak to her since she was at that time on an airplane from Cuernavaca to Dallas to see me. One part flattery and two parts apprehension, I imagined the conversation at the other end. "Oh yes, we're flying up to Dallas to consult a specialist." I also wrote a script based on previous editions which included an overbearing couple expecting red carpets, hot coffee and professional courtesy ("Send that to my insurance company, son"). Not knowing them, I could angle my script to fit any paradigm I liked. This one prepared me for the worst so that disappointment was unlikely. Happily, they didn't read the script. They were special people.

They were in the office at 10AM having flown in the night before and taken a room in town. Lillian, 60 years old, wore a shift like dress, her bare legs thrust into lopsided loafers, grey hair clean but stubborn to the brush. She was pacing about the room with a broad smile and what I thought was nervous energy. Andy got up from his chair as I walked in shook my hand firmly and asked if he could stay. He was a big fellow of girth and muscle. Not intimidating big - warm and friendly big. Lillian insisted that he stay.

"What is the problem?" I asked.

"Well, I just don't know," Lillian, blurted, "It's all so strange and silly."

I looked at Andy expecting him to take charge, as that was how the script read. He looked back at me but said nothing. I looked back at Lillian and several seconds passed. She said no more but continued her brisk walk about the office, touching things, moving them about, straightening the magazines, fiddling with the blinds.

"Do you feel alright?"

"Oh yes perfectly, Doctor."

"Did something happen?"

"Well, yes, I guess it did," she replied. "I was on the phone talking to my sister, and suddenly I couldn't remember what I had said and who I was talking to. Everything sort of went blank and I just hung up. I am so embarrassed!" Another long pause as I waited for more, but there was no more, that was it. Andy smiled gently, chin in palm and added no comment. Lillian giggled and smiled and kept pacing.

How could a dropped phone cause all of this, I wondered? They were perhaps eccentric but not kooks. Get on an airplane and fly to Dallas because of a slip of the memory clutch? "What else was going on at the time of the phone call, Lillian?" I asked.

Again a giggle. "Well, let's see. It was Wednesday, wasn't it Andy? I think it was because on Tuesdays I usually shop. It's not easy to get the fresh vegetables and they usually come in on Tuesdays. There's this very nice outdoor market you see. The melons are so good... Ah, were was I?" snicker and stalk. Andy looked carefully at Lillian then carefully at me but still offered no comment.

"Andy, what do you think happened?" I prodded.

"Just as she said Doctor," he answered.

I wanted to explore Lillian's somewhat strange behavior and affect with Andy but he seemed content that nothing else was worth mentioning. Lillian seemed so light, carefree and ebullient that I became increasingly concerned through the interview that this was a very marked shift in behavior. Andy, I thought, was just too embarrassed to comment.

I finished the physical examination and had jotted only two words on my tablet - suck and snout. Lillian had a suck and snout reflex. Tap her lips with a finger and she would make a sucking pattern of her lips. Tap her on the side of the mouth and she would make the same gesture and move her head like a baby looking for the nipple. The entire remainder of the examination was normal. There was enough however to tell me that there was something very wrong with Lillian's brain. In particular something wrong with her frontal lobes, and specifically her frontal lobes since the rest of her brain seemed okay. This was not dementia. She was wifty all right but not demented. The combination of unusual behavior and the frontal lobe signs bought her a CAT scan of the brain straightaway.

The physical findings had been subtle, the scan was not. It showed a large left frontal lobe tumor almost certainly a malignant primary tumor of the brain. A pewter grey center, which melded into the surrounding swollen brain. They couldn't be seen but surely little tendrils slid along tiny paths around, over and between. I had a new script now. Much more accurate since I really had seen this episode before. It starts with the "Lillian, I am afraid I have some bad news. You have a tumor of the brain." Scene two is the introduction of the need for a tissue diagnosis, that is, an operation. Not just an operation but neurosurgery. Then you ride with the family's hope that this one will be the benign one. Don't argue, don't dissuade, don't agree if pushed, just wait and console when the bad news comes in and give them a plan, give them some decisions to make, give them some facts. Don't sigh. Scene three is the "lets make the best of the time that's left."

I went to the operating room and peered over the neurosurgeon's shoulder. Most people have a vision of neurosurgery as supremely delicate and gentle. It is and it is not. Delicate and gentle in that a small move can wipe out memory, speech, motion, control or life. I find it more gruesome. Start with a scalping in a barber chair. Drill holes spraying bone dust and bits of pink marrow. Connect the dots with a wire saw, grunt and cut. Zap the little bleeders with a cautery, each one recoiling like a singed bug wisping out a tiny tendril of smoke. Blunt dissection with the fingertips and the sucker, always the sucker at hand. It slurps up the soul and spits it into the bottle under the table together with blood, dead tissue, cerebrospinal fluid and any brain not firmly anchored. Not delicate, not delicate at all. Finally, out with Lillian's left frontal lobe. It suddenly seems so small, deflated almost. There is obvious tumor left behind but to take it is mindless.

The fresh wound first viewed in the recovery room is neat and tidy. Two days later, sour and dirty. The crisp red line of the scalp incision turns brown and crusty, the surrounding skin turns green, yellow and blue with bruise and the clean-shaven scalp now has unruly stubble. So it is with the family. A sharp swift stab of death knelling, singular, straight and too huge to let anything else has a comment. Two days later, questions and confusion. "What was the lab report? Will the radiation therapy help a lot? Should we arrange for a home nurse? Any special diet?" The tough questions seem only to come from the distant relatives. Those with enough distance to not be restrained by the thought of bad answers, those with enough distance to only be briefly affected by bad answers, those with enough distance to not need to know the bad answers. "Was there tumor left behind? How long will she live?"

When Lillian recovered enough to sit up in a chair, I searched for some change. I thought of the little glob of her frontal lobe in the stainless steel pan in the operating room and wondered what it contained other than tumor. What part of Lillian went out the sucker or into the pan? I couldn't find anything. Lillian was precisely as she had been in the office. Still laughing, hyperkinetic, euphoric and unconcerned. I assumed the tumor had done maximum damage to the surrounding normal frontal lobe tissue and that its removal had not aggravated her already distorted behavior pattern.

During a quiet time with the family some days later, I said, "Well it looks like Lillian's baseline status is not going to improve."

"What do you mean, Doctor?" asked one of the daughters.

"Well, what I mean is that the change in her affect and behavior is probably not going to go back to the way it was before she got sick," I said.

Now I really had their attention, backs suddenly got straighter and eyes more focused on me. I felt uneasy as if I had spoken the unspeakable. Was the idea of dying of a brain tumor easier to deal with than the warping of the person in the process? No, that was not it at all. What came next was, as the scriptwriters would call 'a dramatic turn'.

"Doctor, I don't know what you're talking about. Lillian's exactly like she has always been. She's always been happy go lucky, energetic and, yes, a little strange but this is nothing new. You see you just never knew her before she got sick!" said Andy.

The epilogue to this little story went on for about nine months and Lillian died. At first, I thought that Lillian was the exception to prove the rule that the best medicine comes when you know the patient. After all, if I had known Lillian, I might have avoided the offense of my gaffe after surgery about her behavior but then if I had known Lillian, I probably would not have made the diagnosis when I did. I would have thought, oh silly Lillian just had a case of phone dropsy, no cause for alarm. Well, I might have felt better about making the quick diagnosis but did Lillian? What would have happened if I had told Lillian and Andy on that first visit that I didn't think much was wrong. Go on back to Quenervaca and don't worry. Of course the tumor would eventually do its dirty deed but might she have had a few more months without worry, a few more fresh peaches on Tuesdays?

Perhaps Lillian was not the exception to the rule. Perhaps my teachers were right.

HEALTH CARE MYTHS

MISCELLANY

In our extensive discussions about health care reform, there are a few oft-repeated statements that don't get the scrutiny they should. Because they are so often repeated they are accepted at face value. Consider the following.

Myth: More preventive medicine would save health care costs. There are many good reasons to support preventive medicine but saving health care costs is not one of them. In fact one of the reasons health care is so expensive is because prevention has been successful. I did not die at age 8 of polio. As a consequence, I have had an additional 60 years of health care costs and I will likely die of heart disease, cancer, stroke or complications of Alzheimer's disease – all very costly. Mortality is still 100% and unlikely to go lower. There is one area where prevention can save health care costs and that is in secondary prevention. We can save medicine by preventing some of the complications of chronic disease for instance. If the diabetic is prevented from blindness, dialysis or limb amputation there is money to be saved.

Myth: Health care consumes 17% of the Gross Domestic Product. This is false because you cannot consume the GDP. It is the sum of all goods and services in our economy. By using the term "consume" we suggest that absent health care there would be this great piece of pie that could otherwise go to the economy. In fact absent health care millions of jobs would be lost; pharmaceuticals, device manufacturers, research institutions and the like would be forfeit. There is nothing that says that a society should not so value health care as to devote 17% of its energies on it. If you would like to shrink health care as a percentage of the GDP you can either grow the rest of the economy at a greater rate or reduce by artificial means the expenditures on health.

Myth: There are 45 million people without health care. There are 45 million people without health care insurance. They are in fact, receiving health care not the best perhaps but they are being cared for. They appear in doctor's offices and the emergency rooms of the country. Doctor's still give care at no cost and emergency rooms must take care of them by law. It is difficult to follow the dollar but some of it is property tax as in Tarrant County, some by charitable organizations, a lot by cost shifting meaning that what you pay for health care subsidizes those who have no health insurance. If you have health insurance, part of your premium is used to support Medicaid and Medicare patients and part to subsidize the uninsured. The point is that to provide care to the uninsured is less than you might think. It is the usual annual cost of health care minus that which is already being spent. The problem will be the unraveling of the bizarre way the money currently flows.

Myth: Technology has escalated health care costs. Technology is all of the drugs and devices used in health care from stethoscopes to MRIs. Much of this technology has in fact reduced the costs of health care. Diagnostic accuracy has improved, invasive procedures are now non-invasive and hospital stays have been reduced. The increase in cost is because the threshold for using these technologies has gone lower and lower. It doesn't cost the patient that much and is proded by our risk aversion society.

Myth: You can increase the number of people cared for and reduce health care costs and maintain the level of care at the same time. Something has to give.

BAG BALM

HERSHEY

I came to the Hershey Medical Center shortly after clinical services began. Prior to the construction of this medical college, Hershey was well served by the ministrations of several family physicians. There were specialists to be seen in Harrisburg and Baltimore, but for the most part Hershey illness was treated by Hershey doctors.

Now, however we were in town and we were a "major medical center" as the press would have it. Never mind that the entire department of medicine numbered just ten physicians. We couldn't even dissuade the White House when President Nixon made a sweep through central Pennsylvania and they designated us the "nearest facility to which the Chief Executive was to be taken in the event of unforeseen circumstance." When the hospital first opened to receive patients, the chiefs of medicine, surgery and pediatrics - in shifts, staffed the emergency room. Gratefully, no one "circumstanced" the President.

We were lean at the edges and didn't really feel major medical then. My lofty title was Chief, Division of Internal Medicine - a one-man division. Major subspecialties were covered - cardiology, endocrinology, oncology, hematology and gastro-enterology. Many of the others fell to me and my division of me.

"You need a rheumatologist?" the operator would query. "Perhaps you will be well served to begin with one of our general internists", she would gently suggest. And so, I got the arthritis patients, the pulmonary patients and, ouch, the dermatology patients.

Fresh from residency training and fully prepared through my requisite month to six-week rotations on the above specialties, I masqueraded as the local expert. After all, I was trained in Boston and was bringing all the knowledge of the modern western world to terra incognita.

A really fine library and a little black book of phone numbers of my mentors in different disciplines rescued me from sure disaster on several occasions. I felt some confidence in knowing what I did know and what I did not know and had a sweaty palmed sense of when I was in over my head. On several occasions, it was the patient himself who managed the sorting out.

This was the case with Roland Anspach. A fine no-nonsense local farmer. Roland had lived in the area all of his life and took over the farm when his father passed away. He was all sinews and creases - very lean and very quiet. He milked forty dairy cattle and tilled about 200 acres.

Roland was sent by a local family physician because of a stubborn rash.

"Doc Henry said to see you. Said you was the expert on rashes."

I hoped that there wasn't quite as much disbelief in his statement as I thought I heard and in my most professorial manner said, "Well, let's take a look, Mr. Anspach. I've seen quite a few rashes".

He took off his cotton gloves and I stared at two raw hamburger patties. The skin of both hands was torn, lifted, weeping and blood red. I had never seen anything like it. Covering my astonishment with some learned statement like, "Hmm, how long have they been this way"? I also noted that Roland was tolerating the obvious pain stoically. A bright light and a small magnifying lens bought me some time but no inkling of the nature of the malady.

"Excuse me for a minute, Roland, I have to take a call", allowed me to escape to the back office and the standard texts. The best that I could reason was that since it was confined to his hands and had a reasonably sudden onset a few weeks ago that a) it was probably a contact dermatitis and b) most importantly, probably would not be fatal.

"Roland, that sure looks like some kind of allergic reaction. I want you to use some of this cream under gloves at night. I also want you to bring me a list of all the solvents, fertilizers and chemicals you use on the farm. Think carefully about any that you used for the first time when this all started." Writing with a pen that I wished was a magic marker, I whisked off a prescription and arranged to see him in a week.

I noticed some improvement when he returned. At least some of the inflammation was better but the cracks and peeling continued. This time I was ready. Scrapings - I will get some scrapings, heat under a little potassium hydroxide and see if I could identify some branching organisms of the yeast and fungus family. Was that skin flakes, dust or maybe hyphae that I saw under the microscope?

"Could be there is a little infection on top of that allergic reaction, Roland. Best we add some antibiotics to that steroid cream. That aught to do the trick." Roland evinced more hope than I felt and left with a new prescription and another appointment.

Over the subsequent weeks, I think we went through the entire dermatologic pharmacopoeia including an unfair bout of gentian violet. The latter did little except to bring a complaint from Mrs. Anspach that the damn stuff stains everything. Blood tests, cultures and a small skin biopsy only ran up Roland's bill and ran down his patience.

Then it happened. Roland appeared with nearly completely healed hands. Healthy new skin was growing in, the cracks were closed and the color near normal.

"That was really stubborn, Roland, but at least that last medicine seems to be doing the trick", I declared with a great sense of relief and triumph.

"Well Doc, let me tell you. I threw your stuff away and started using some stuff I had at home."

"What stuff Roland?" I asked crestfallen.

"Bag Balm."

"What did you use?"

"You know, Bag Balm", in a what you dummy tone. "Here, I brought you some so you'd have it around in case you need it for someone else", he said handing me a small square tin.

The lid was brightly decorated with a smiling cow - yes a smiling cow wreathed with a garland of roses. The careful lettering on the side contended "... for minor abrasions and irritations of the teats. Proven for generations. Apply once daily. Sold at reputable feed stores everywhere."

We laughed together and I assured Roland that I would share his discovery with others and I thanked him. He left with a smile and a warm handshake - the first since he'd been to see me.

BACK OF THE LIBRARY

MISCELLANY

I went to the back of the library today. I stop in the library probably three times a week. Usually, it is fifteen minutes or so between meetings, appointments or before or after lunch. I guess I developed a routine without really knowing it. I would go to the new releases section of the journals to find the issues which are new, scan some tables of contents, read a few abstracts, maybe a full article and if really impressed run a photocopy of some great tidbit to take back to my office, file carefully then never read again.

I've always been heavy on the top of the alphabet and concentrate on the front of the library - Archives to Journal of ... only occasionally getting into the Morbidities and Neurons. Today for some reason I strode confidently into the unknown passing my comfortable Annals of Internal Medicine, past the American Journal of Medicine and the Journal of the American Medical Association, deeper and deeper in the stacks till I found the source - Xenobiotica.

Xenobiotica the title - the subtitle read, The Fate of Foreign Compounds in Biological Systems. Nearby stood Vox Sanguinis - An International Journal of Transfusion Medicine. I move up through Trauma, and Transfusion to Theta Thymus, the Journal of Thymology to the Tokushima Journal of Experimental Medicine whose editors remind authors that they might have to pay to have fancy pictures or graphs included in their articles. Then I found the Philosophical Transactions of the Royal Society of London, a title of great appeal. Visions of a foggy London night, a good meal, brandy and cigars followed by a scholarly presentation and conversation about a weighty subject. Science the old fashioned way.

The volume felt promising - the cover was a simple tan colored half cardboard and the paper inside cheap in quality. The entire issue was devoted to a 57-page monograph entitled "An Allometric Study of Pulmonary Morphometric Parameters in Birds, with Mamalian Comparisons." The authors, one from Nairobi and two from Liverpool must have had a fascinating collaboration to sustain such a distance and such a remote research topic. It pointed out also the difference between British and European biomedical research and that conducted in the U.S. Over there, a life's work might appear in a single monograph whereas we are so driven to have quick results that we would chop up the results in six-monthly bites to be published fifteen times.

Next I found Placenta and Plasmid, A Journal Focused on Extrachromosomal Gene Systems. Many of these Journals extolled that they were "International Journals". Perhaps that is the only way they can find a sufficient audience for what seemed to be rather obscure topics. It certainly seemed to be a signal to an outrageous annual subscription fee of $250 plus for many of these International offerings.

I moved from the splitters focused on single organs or cells to the lumpers who seek to combine and find links - Suicide and Life Threatening Behavior and PsychoNeuroEndocrinology (also International in scope).

Next my eye fell on a most beautiful journal - The Quarterly Review of Biology. The stock was a rich cream-colored paper and the cover had lovely red icons around the border. The typeface was very important appearing as it explained "The Maintenance of Species Diversity by Disturbance".

As I drifted back to the comfort of mid-alphabet, I was struck that I had found in each of these obscure issues some small tidbit of interest and potential use for the treatment of patients in the clinic or hospital.

How much more must there be in all the bound journals and texts, which I could find useful? If I stayed in here forever could I get it all and not make any mistakes out there?

DESERTED ISLAND

MISCELLANY

I have a fantasy about a deserted island. This island is temperate, well provisioned with water, fruits, and vegetables and perhaps good fishing. A safe place but no communications, no people, perhaps a dog or goat and no way off save by a visiting ship once a twelvemonth.

In this fantasy, I have control of the residency requirements and the passenger manifest of the visiting steamer. I can write the pre-scription, which reads:

Rx: One deserted island

One year

Sig: As directed

No refills

While I'm at it, and since this is fantasy, let me have as many of these islands as needed since I will have trouble were I forced to choose among the many who might benefit. Such a prescription could be life giving, perhaps life saving. A kind of Statue of Liberty for the weak, tired and dizzy, for the yearning souls eager to be co-cooned lest they break or dissolve, for those certain that life cannot be lived absent pills, lotions, potions or salves.

"Oh Doctor, I'm so tired..."

"Doctor, I just know it glandular..."

"Don't you have some pills to give me pep..."?

"I just know something is seriously wrong..." (For the complaint of twelve years duration.)

"If only I didn't have this (headache, backache, abdominal pain, neck pain, fatigue...), I'm sure I could (work, graduate, keep my wife, succeed, love, move...)

I don't dislike these patients and I'm not really angry but I do get frustrated when the obvious isn't. We, as doctors, take the easy way out. There's always one more test, one more pill or one more specialist to see. We are so afraid of not treating something that might be there that we will treat something that is not there. We overdo everything except honesty. Having tried to convince the world that if anything is wrong "see your Doctor", we're surprised that they see us when anything is wrong. If the patient thinks he has a medical problem and we don't, do anything but don't argue the point. It's hard to do and we could be mistaken. Suppose that headache of twelve years really is a brain tumor? We laugh nervously at the joke of the epitaph on the psychosomatics grave that reads, "See, I told you I was sick!"

Treating no disease is rather like paddling with a fork - it takes lots of energy and you don't get very far. It's not really hard to diagnose no disease. Take any ten clinicians, give them a ten minute case presentation and within three minutes they've tumbled to the diagnosis of no disease. Oh yes, they'll dance at the edges a bit with, "Did you consider Lyme disease, ...chronic EB virus infection, ...click murmur (forme fruste of course)". This is just to play the game and keep the options open for the rare, "I thought there was something a little fishy here." All of our training compels us to find the physical explanation for any dis-ease when a lot of heart pain is really heart-ache. It's not hard to diagnose but very difficult to treat.

"Mrs. Brown, I understand your abdominal pain. It is very real and I know a great worry to you. Fortunately, all of the tests exclude a life threatening illness. There is no evidence of cancer of any incurable disease.

"Let's try to understand what's going on. I think your stomach is your Achilles' heel - kind of a weak spot that talks to you first whenever things aren't quite right in your life. Everyone has such a weak spot. For some people its headaches, for others their blood pressure or an ulcer or diarrhea and so on. The feeling is real, not for a moment imagined. What we really need to get at is the cause. Think of life stress as a fist full of energy. When we don't spend that energy mentally, it comes out physically.

"Now, what I want you to do is re-interpret your pain. When you get it I want you to say, 'Ah, there's my friend telling me something is not right in my life'. When you put your finger on the trigger and deal with the problems bothering you, your pain will get better."

"You mean to say this is all in my head?" is the usual incredulous retort. "But, ...but Dr. Jones said my serum porcupine level was borderline and. and what about this bloating? Can't you see it?" now close to tears.

Once in a while the response goes like this.

"Doctor, I think I understand. You mean when I have pain it means that I'm under stress or there's something bothering me that I haven't worked out? There's really nothing seriously wrong? Boy, I feel better already. That's wonderful."

And then... and then, hand on the doorknob, the head turns over the shoulder and you hear, "Doc, what about the headaches I told you about shouldn't we check them out too?"

That's when my fantasy takes over. Let me have my island. Deposit this soul there for a year. Let him know he's not dying, not fragile. Her body is strong and resilient. He can be self sufficient, as brave as need be. The dog and goat won't answer the whines or change because of her pain. There's adequate rain without his tears. A back to basics course of building a shelter, slaking a thirst and gathering some food.

I'll bet this prescription will work better than some others I've written.

DOCTORING DOCTORS

HERSHEY

I have two rules for taking care of doctors. The first rule is to do everything the usual way. Do not cut corners or try to 'expedite' anything. The reason we have routines is that they work best. Change the routine and you invite trouble. The second rule is to assume that a doctor patient knows nothing at all about medicine. Doctors as teachers have been important to me but doctors as patients have taught me even more.

Paul Levy, M.D. was a special doctor patient teacher. I think of him often - often with sadness but more often with gratitude. He didn't come to see me, I was summoned to see him and a friendship of many years began.

Dr. Levy was hospitalized on the cardiology service with a complaint of severe chest pain and palpitations. He was in the coronary care unit and the orders were routine "R/O Myocardial Infarction" orders. For some providential reason, the admitting resident had included a sedimentation rate in the battery of laboratory tests. The Prince of Serendip visited and the test came back markedly elevated. Now, a sedimentation rate is exquisitely sensitive but not very specific. It is likely to be elevated in very many conditions but it tells little about the specific condition it is responding to.

The chief of cardiology was kind to me. I was a new faculty member, had an interest in rheumatology and immunology and I guess I didn't look overworked so he asked me to opine about this curious finding.

It was mid-afternoon when I met Paul Levy and I liked him immediately. He had passed fifty-eight birthdays. He was portly with the kind of bulk that suggested great physical strength. He had a wreath of grey hair around central baldness and wire rimmed glasses framing clear blue eyes. He spoke very softly and made no hand gestures other than twinning his large fingers lightly tapping his thumbs together. There were few clues in the room. I like to look for clues - a copy of Hans Kung and Sports Afield on the night stand, a standard hospital gown (no silk pajamas), a small vase of hand picked flowers and a few get well cards.

I was at first nervous but he quickly put me at ease. He was pleased to see me and the next hour went fast. The questions, answers and examination led me to the diagnosis - a good diagnosis - not spectacular but fine. Paul had, I was sure, giant cell arteritis and polymyalgia rheumatica. That's a mouthful (a sure characteristic of known diseases with unknown causes). It is a diagnosis that will occur to any rheumatologist when faced with a patient mid to late aged with a very high sedimentation rate. His positive responses to aches in the shoulders and hips, fevers, weight loss and mild anemia were all characteristic of this curious illness. His chest pain was probably because of inflammation of his coronary blood vessels and did not represent atherosclerosis at all. Well, it was one thing to let the new kid on the block give it a shot but quite another to abide by the startling recommendations offered. High dose corticosteroids are not in the pharmacopaeia of cardiologists and did I really mean to say that the precious pre- ordained protocol for chest pain was to be abandoned?

"Give him forty milligrams of prednisone for three days and he'll thank you," I said with more confidence than I really felt.

They did and he did. The rest of the hospitalization was brief. The cardiologists sort of wiped their hands of him since he didn't really fit. Grudgingly, I suspect, they arranged for him to see me in my office for follow up two weeks later. His improvement had been dramatic which in this illness tends to confirm the diagnosis. He presented me with a basket of fresh picked apples and wonderful conversation. There was a little shyness as he let me know who he was. The medical center had intimidated him a bit, it seemed. Paul Levy had for years been a practitioner in Ephrata - a little town resistant to the incursions of nearby Reading and the corridor leading to Philadelphia - home of the Cloisters, Amish, Mennonites and other self sufficients. His specialty was homeopathy - about which I know very little. He began to teach me, not with evangelism but with little tests of information as if to see my reaction and was it safe to tell me more or would I scoff at his quiet catechism? I was curious about this theory of medicine. The basic tenet, I learned, was that medicinals, which produced symptoms that the patient complained of, would be therapeutic when given in very small doses. The idea had been around for years and was generally scoffed at by the scientists since there were no data to confirm it.

Paul rarely hospitalized patients himself preferring to refer them to the staff at the local hospitals. His clientele was astounding. Devoted patients would travel long distances for his counsel, advice and remedies. Science or not he helped many through difficult times with his care. Perhaps it was the remedies and perhaps he fit the expectations of patients who trusted the earth and her plants. He shunned antibiotics and detail salesmen. He knew when a remedy was not in his jars and vials and gently suggested a referral to a more traditionally oriented doctor. He worked long hours with pleasure, taking time out to go home to eat dinner or supper and do an occasional chore at his nearby farm. We continued visiting in my office for perhaps two years. His disease required attention although he could have done it himself; as many doctors are want to do. I believe he enjoyed our chats as much as I did. Stubbornly, his polymyalgia refused to remit completely although we were able to reduce the dose of prednisone to small amounts sufficient to control his symptoms and not give him side effects of this powerful remedy.

One day I received a handwritten note inviting my family to Sunday dinner at his farm. We packed up, admonished the boys to be on good behavior and drove to Ephrata. He lived off the main highway on a narrow macadam road. It was late August and the road was a pleasant tunnel through high lush green corn fields. The Levy home was a fine large stone farmhouse close sided to the road with a large porch around three sides. The broad well-worn entrance was to the kitchen not the front door as is the custom in farm homes. The stone was carefully pointed, window frames crisp white and the large neat stone barn showed signs of a working farm. The inside of the house showed love of history. It was not a home that had been restored. It was rather a home that had been maintained for generations.

We visited around the kitchen table meeting his wife. She was his second wife, his first having died at a young age. Two grown children, we were told, were living away but would be home for Christmas. Had we been farm laborers the meal would have been quite sufficient. For us it was hearty to pleasant discomfort. Our wives tidied in the kitchen, the boys went to explore the barn and Paul and I went to a picnic table in the orchard to drink coffee and talk. Shafts of late afternoon sun slipped through the trees on one of those rare crystal clear fall days. One of those visions that you are not really conscious of at the moment but which sticks to you in later years.

He looked at his watch and said he had a late patient coming to the office and would I like to come along? The invitation was a special gift and I was happy to accept. His office was a converted house on the main street. As he talked with his patient in his consultation office, I explored the other rooms. The office showed the same care as the home. No stainless steel or plastic here. Warm woods and antique ladder back chairs in the waiting room. One large room was the apothecary. Mahogany boxes, glass vials of different shapes and sizes and a strange admixture of pleasant unidentifiable odors. Each container was hand labeled with the same hand I had seen on the invitation to visit. In the back room I found a strange item. A very very old black x-ray machine and fluoroscope. It looked to be Roentgen's original machine and there was a small darkroom next to it.

During his exposition of the remedies he used, I casually asked him about the x-ray. "Oh yes," he said, "I take lots of x-rays and even do some contrast studies. I got interested in it many years ago and it's sort of a side hobby of mine. I never charge for them." Now, I know only a little about homeopathy but I do know something about radiation and I was alarmed but not to the point of mentioning anything. I should have.

About a year later, Paul called and related complaints that he and I both concluded sounded like thrombophlebitis of his left leg. He came to the office and indeed had deep phlebitis in the calf and up into the groin. I insisted on immediate hospitalization so that we could anticoagulate him with heparin. The bad news call came from the laboratory shortly after admission. Paul's white blood cell count was 42,000 with many immature forms and circulating blast cells. The morphology was that of myelomonocytic leukemia. The mahogany boxes and dried leaves of his world gave way to the poisons and chemistries of my world in a desperate challenge to beat this almost uniformly fatal disease. He vomited continuously, bled from low platelets and became septic with bacteria. Two weeks of induction therapy and misery and not much change except that we were destroying most of his marrow - good and bad bone marrow.

Then one morning during my visit he seemed strangely distracted and agitated. Things had just begun to improve. His blood counts had bottomed out and his fever had lysed the day before. To this point he had been quite attentive to his illness and the treatment but not that morning.

"John," he said. "Listen carefully. This is important. I had a vision last night."

"A vision?"

"Yes, yes a vision. Not a dream, a vision. I was wide-awake.
Now, I'm not a very religious person but something happened that I couldn't explain. I... I feel blessed!"

I was dumb. I fear I looked at him with an open mouthed gape. This was Paul, my friend - quiet, honest and thoughtful, not some mystic with flashes of fancy.

"Tell me about it, Paul."

"I saw myself sitting in a large easy chair. I was holding a small lamb. The lamb was bleating and then started to bleed in my arms and it died. I felt cleansed and relieved! There was a wonderful peace as if.. as if everything will be alright."

The scientist me concluded that this must have been delirium from fever, intense sickness, drugs, septicemia - all of it. Another part of me wondered. I know medicine to be good science but I have also learned that medicine is magic and mystery. Most magic and mystery becomes science when it is explained but still some persists unexplained. I didn't know what to make of all this but whatever it was, Paul went into remission from his leukemia and was discharged from the hospital.

He was at peace and even more quiet and reflective than before. He knew, and we talked about, the inevitability of a relapse. He would have no second course of treatment he told me. He had been given a "God gift" he called it and planned to use this time to prepare his family, his friends, his patients, his office staff and most especially himself. He would ask for no more, he said.

The remission lasted for six months and Paul died at home in peace without discomfort. I still think about orchards in late summer, about lambs and about ugly, black, leaky, x-ray machines.

GEORGE AND JOSEPHINE

HERSHEY

George was a giant. George was also very sick, very near death when I first met him in the emergency room. His six foot six frame extended over the end of the litter. I lost my hand in his palm. Two hundred fifty pounds seemed slapped on his huge frame but it was not a proportionate fit. His arms and legs were longer than they should have been. He had large floppy ears, great fleshy folds on his face, thick bifocal lenses, a pigeon breast and very flat feet. The parts were ugly but the whole was impressive. He was gray green in color, there was a sheen of sweat on his brow and he was afraid. Angor animi - death was near and George knew it and so did I. He was complaining of chest pain - a great tearing pain beneath his breast and into his back between his shoulder blades.

It was not hard to diagnose what was happening to George. He had never heard of Dr. Marfan but Dr. Marfan, a French physician of a previous century had known George or at least George's kindred. George had Marfan's syndrome. This syndrome is a disease of connective tissue, the scaffolding web around which we build our organs. Fibrous tissue, elastic tissue and collagen, a kind of rubbery glue around and between which we construct the engines of life. Instead of being strong and flexible, George's connective tissue was flawed - it was lax and brittle. His growth had been distorted by this lack of a firm blueprint and now he had the most feared complication of the disease. His aorta was ripping apart. A small tear had begun in the wall of this largest of all arteries in the body. The tear started just as this vessel leaves the heart. The pounding column of blood finds the tear and lifts the flap and burrows underneath splitting the wall. Now there are two channels instead of one - the normal one leading to supply the vital organs and a false one leading nowhere. As the nowhere channel enlarges, it chokes off the vital one. The false channel either breaks through the outside of the wall of the aorta with a fatal burst of the dam or it breaks back into the normal channel. The diagnosis is easy but the treatment is not. The surgeons nodded and withdrew.

I went to the waiting room to find George's wife. Scanning the worried and bored I almost missed her. I was looking for a likely match not the tiny little wisp at the periphery of my vision.

"Mrs. Stark..."

"Call me Josie."

"Josie, your husband is very ill," I said, hating this way of meeting someone - draping crepe.

"Yes, I know," she said gently. "I knew that when he woke up with such pain. Don't worry doctor, he'll be alright. He's so strong."

She was actually comforting me! My surprise was dual. I was surprised at her response and surprised by looking at her. Josie was as small as George was large. Tiny and childlike, she looked old and young at the same time. She had alabaster skin and very blue eyes which graced a somewhat plain face.

The King's Horses and the King's Men swirled about shortly after admission and it was decided to "manage conservatively", which means sit and wait. We controlled his blood pressure and kept George quiet. George's pain continued but moved slowly down his back and into the pit of his stomach as the dissection continued. The pulse in his left groin became weak as the false channel squeezed the great vessel to his leg.

Josie set up vigil in George's room. Not an hysterical vigil, not even a seriously worried vigil, more a presence. They talked quietly, never to be overheard, and occasionally shared a small laugh. We came in for rounds, Josie would quickly stand and move against the wall, a shy smile on her face. We felt we were in her home and she was a simple gracious hostess.

On the third day, George suddenly had relief of his pain and his leg pulse became strong again. He had re-entered the main channel. Josie smiled tolerantly at our elation. She seemed a little critical of our previous doubts that George would survive. By great good fortune, the tear in his aorta had spiraled along its length without shearing off any major branches. There remained the chance that George would develop a new tear but he had survived this one and went home taking medication to keep his blood pressure low and admonitions to avoid heavy labor. He expected the later advice and I expected he would not follow it.

Over the next six months, George and Josie reported regularly to the office and their mutual affection became even clearer. He returned to work hauling engine blocks, grunting with torque wrenches and contorting his huge frame under and around automobiles. Josie knew this was bad medicine but she also knew George. Rather than nag or cajole, she supported him making it easy for him to rest when she could. She knew that no work was more deadly than what he was doing and she accepted it gladly. George showed equal concern for his bride. His manners with this tiny woman were courtship like in common ways and thoughtful in uncommon ways. He nodded at her near whispered comments and suggestions.

On one visit they both appeared solemn and resolved. They had reached a decision and prepared mutually to inform me. They had decided that I should now attend to Josie. The gravity with which they made this request should have alerted me but I missed the gesture's significance.

Josie had few physical complaints, some easy fatigue, dispersed aches and pains, an occasional headache, dizziness once in a while and a rare bout of palpitations. I asked about her menstrual and sexual history and got a blunt, "You'll see".

Indeed, I did see. Disrobed and in a hospital gown for a physical examination, I discovered the reason for Josie's 'old-young' appearance. Josie had never sexually matured. She had never gone through puberty. She had no breasts and no genital maturation. Josie was virginal and childlike. Startling findings like this really rattle an internist's bone box. Internists love puzzles especially when they are the first to encounter them. I had to hold myself from a rapid fire cascade of questions to get to the bottom of this puzzle. Josie looked me straight in the eye waiting for my response. She was not fearful nor embarrassed, just expectant. I held my tongue.

"Thank you, Josie. You can get dressed now."

I worried over what to do. Some delicate switch in Josie never closed years ago. Should we try to bring menarche to a woman of fifty-eight? Breasts are important, orgasms are important, woman-ness is important - important for everybody. Important for Josie? Even if Josie couldn't mourn the loss of something she had never had wasn't there some bitterness that she had been denied the substance of so much art, literature and story. Yet, this was my mind at work. I was a well meaning but perhaps sinister 'If I were you, I would have it differently'. From all of this natural misadventure, Josie wrested happiness, devotion, hospitality and love.

"What shall we do about your condition, Josie?"

"Am I sick, Doctor?", she replied with a little smile.

"Well, not sick, Josie but not normal either as you surely know."

"Oh yes, Doctor. I know I am not normal as does George but I feel well and we are happy", she said.

A disease but not a dis-ease. A few laboratory tests confirmed that it was not a threat either. The remaining functions of her pituitary gland were normal and there was no slowly growing tumor. When they both knew this they were content and decided to come back to see me only if in need.

The need didn't arise until a few years later when Josie burst a blood vessel in her brain. She nearly died as the hemorrhage flooded her left brain taking away her speech and all motion on the right side and left her in a wheelchair. Her communication was a series of inflective "na, na, na, na". With this single syllable and about an octave of tones, Josie could be understood by George who tended her with the same care that he had received. She still seemed happy. It seems to me that basic dispositions are preserved in people who have strokes. Mean and ugly people tend to become more so and basically happy people remain so when the controlling brain cortex is destroyed.

Josie progressively declined and died and George went into profound mourning. He came to see me only to weep and re-examine the details looking for reassurance that we had done all we could. Did we do everything? Are you sure she wasn't in pain? His only forward thought was for his own death.

"It won't be much longer will it Doctor?"

It wasn't.

DIRECTORY OF MEDICAL SPECIALTIES

MISCELLANY

CARDIOLOGY
    The bundle of Hiss is small
    but you can make a career of it
    or Syncopated syncope

EMERGENCY MEDICINE
    Phone booth and cape
    junkies

ENDOCRINOLOGY
    Feedback loop, loop, loop

GENERAL SURGERY
    Skin to skin
    Real quick

GASTRO-ENTEROLOGY
    Through the gut with
    gun and camera

INTERNAL MEDICINE
    Thoughtful
    Articulate
    Ineffective

INTENSIVISTS
    Apache warriors

NEUROLOGY
    Soul strokers

NEUROSURGERY
    Inflation
    leads to
    Depression

JOHN W. BURNSIDE, M.D.

OBSTETRICS AND GYNECOLOGY
Stirrups and spurs
Autonomy saddled

OPHTHALMOLOGY
Soul voyeurs

ORTHOPEDICS
Big he's
Few she's

PEDIATRICS
Pacifiers

PLASTIC SURGERY
Nip and tuck
in the nick of time

PSYCHIATRY
In it for themselves

UROLOGY
Chips and dips(ticks)

KATHERINE AND SAMANTHA

DALLAS

Katherine McCoy was a third year medical student when I met her. I was the teaching attending at Parkland Memorial Hospital and she was one of the students on our team of three students, one intern and one junior resident. These teams work hard together and I have found it helpful to me to know about the students and residents before starting a new rotation. I review their student folders or their residency applications. Who comes from the mid-west, who plays the flute, which did well on previous rotations, who was the oldest in a big family?

Katherine was from a background of special wealth, education, manners and dress. Her family was prominent citizens of Abilene; most of her education had been at private schools where she had done very well. There was a long list of extra-curricular activities and student honors. Meeting her confirmed all this and more. You could not help noticing Katherine. She somehow made you sit up straighter and speak more precisely. Her clothes, Gucci pumps, and perfect makeup had no aspect of affectation; it just went with the person. She was neither intimidating nor arrogant just a nice non-verbal reminder that if we tried just a bit harder we could be better people. Even without these trappings, she would still be recognized as a beautiful woman - an observation made by all of us. Because of these things we sometimes forgot that she was just as junior as her student colleagues and that she had the same insecurities and uncertainties about clinical medicine.

This was her first clinical rotation, the first real laying on of hands and I worried that Parkland would be a shock. To be sick and poor amounts to more than the sum. Frustration, anger, humiliation and ignorance quickens the rot of disease and when the disease gets to Parkland, it's often late and desperate. Delicate conversation and mild manners might appear professional but to many Parkland patients it is interpreted as condescending. Katherine was in foreign territory. Parkland patients had never appeared on her dance card. It was almost like having a coming out party at a downtown Greyhound bus station. The first night of call could sting her enthusiasm for medicine. The residents were too busy to be worried - more meat for the Parkland mill. As it turned out, I was the one being condescending and unnecessarily paternalistic.

We gathered the next morning after that first night of call to review the patients admitted the previous twenty-four hours. Katherine presented her first patient.

"Samantha Brown is a 23 year old black intravenous drug user admitted with shaking chills and fever. She was well until the day of admission when she had the onset of severe chills, nausea, weakness and a fever to 104 degrees. She shoots daily cocaine and has previously been admitted with fever thought, after full evaluations, to be an allergic reaction."

What an introduction to clinical medicine. "Shooters" with fever are commonplace at Parkland. Frequently it means infected heart valves, a long hospital stay and dubious outcome. If I could have arranged it, Katherine would have been given some nice grandmother with diabetes and a little heart failure. A toe in the water rather than a cannonball.

"Okay", I said. "Tell me the rest", noting that she seemed nonplussed. In fact she looked better than her fellow students who were grey-green after a sleepless night, packed in rumpled scrub suits and scuffed Reeboks. Katherine looked great.

"Well, she couldn't give much history", Katherine said, "since she was delirious. On physical examination, her blood pressure was 90/60, pulse 120, and temperature 104. There was a soft systolic murmur along the left sternal border, rhonchi in both lung fields, some tenderness in the lower abdomen and large ulcers over the dorsum of both wrists. Other than the delirium, the neurologic examination was normal and non-focal."

She continued with the laboratory evaluation. "The hematocrit was 33%, the white blood cell count 22,000 with a shift to the left and the rest of the blood work was normal. The chest films showed bilateral patchy infiltrates and a slightly enlarged heart. The electrocardiogram was normal. We did a lumbar puncture which was normal."

It was a very concise presentation. Katherine knew we had seven patients to review. She was pleased to lead off but didn't steal time from her colleagues. "Let's go see her", I suggested.

The processional into the room was to the strains of "Good Morning America" on the overhead T.V. probably more for the attendants who went in and out than for either of the patients in the room. Samantha was not to be seen. All we could see was a long log covered with twisted blankets. We peeled some away to find her head. She averted her eyes and looked off to the floor. Samantha had a marine crew cut and there was a sheen of sweat on her forehead. When she did dart a look at us there was a flash of startling white sclera and white teeth. Startling against her very black skin - undiluted black, purple black.

"She's better this morning", volunteered Katherine trying to break Samantha's silence to our greeting. "Her temperature is down and she's oriented now. She still complained early this morning about some abdominal pain and nausea".

I continued the unveiling. There were indeed the findings of a murmur, bilateral pneumonia, and two large ugly weeping ulcers on the backs of her wrists. These were desperation ports since all other veins in her arms and legs were reduced to knotted strings from repeated injections. In spite of all this, the veil couldn't hide the fact that Samantha was a beautiful woman and sensuous even in her distress. While I continued my examination, the rest of the team adopted the Parkland slouch - leaning against the walls, foot up on a chair, scribbling on the scutwork board and fighting fatigue. All but Katherine. She watched Samantha intently, occasionally flicking her gaze at me. She seemed tense even perhaps afraid. There was little conversation with Samantha. Yes was a grunt and no a wag of the head. We retired to the hall to wrap up.

Our working diagnosis was bacterial endocarditis of the right side of the heart, which had sent infected debris from the heart valve to her lungs. The blood cultures would probably be positive and in the meantime she was getting appropriate antibiotics. An echocardiogram was scheduled for later in the morning and the cultures might be out that afternoon. We moved on.

Over the next few days our suppositions were confirmed. The blood cultures were positive and we began to learn a little more about Samantha. "Does she work at night?" I asked one day trying to be careful with my diction and what I presumed were delicate sensitivities.

"Oh no", said Katherine, "she doesn't have a regular job. She's a prostitute and has been since she was twelve." So much for delicate sensitivities.

"What about her abdominal pain and nausea?" I asked.

"Still a problem", said Katherine. "We did an abdominal x-ray which was negative. She seems worse in the morning. Lots of pain and lethargy but she improves during the day."

Now there was a familiar verse. "Does her man visit her at night?"

"You mean her pimp?" asked Katherine.

"Yes, sometimes they sneak in and shoot up their girls. Check that out and also let's get an ultrasound of her abdomen to see whether she might have a tubal abscess or something else giving her pain."

The next day brought a heavy dose of embarrassment and contemplation. Samantha, it turned out, was pregnant. The ultrasound showed an eight to nine week fetus. Heads were down and toes scuffed the tile. We were all astonished that a condition for which Samantha was so much at risk should have been discounted at the outset. Somehow we all assumed that a prostitute could not, would not get pregnant. The combination of cocaine, bacteremia, potent antibiotics and abdominal x-rays made it unlikely that this would be a successful pregnancy. Katherine suffered more than her fair share of our collective guilt. Samantha said, "No mind. Lost the last three. Gonna lose this one." She did, about one week later.

As the days passed, Samantha improved. What I had first interpreted as arrogance and anger proved to really be an intense shyness. In her world to be shy was to invite brutality. Protection came only from a costume of strength. She used many disguises. The crew cut, we learned, was to accommodate a variety of wigs or for those who liked their sex "kinky". The unveiling which began that first morning continued as the cocaine washed out and good food took its place. Samantha showed ever-greater beauty.

Katherine and Samantha seemed to circle each other closer and closer. On two occasions while walking past her room, I could see them talking together. Heads close, short laugh, long pause, a few words, an affirmative nod by one or the other. It was a curious private alchemy and I could only speculate. It seemed to be two women each aware of the other's beauty and perhaps each in awe of the others life experiences. Not opposites more like anagrams. Katherine of the cold cream and Samantha of the semen.

I and, I suspect the rest of our team - all men - felt to be intruders. On rounds, Katherine became the conversant with Samantha and was in close while the rest of us held back.

They seemed to be answering for each other and shared the determination to get Samantha well and out of the hospital. Katherine showed courage and she will be a fine physician.

She did get well and was discharged after a long hospital stay. After many months, I still think about this episode and what it taught me. I think I learned that as a teacher I could be honest without being brutal and empathetic without being paternal. It was also a reminder that teaching means taking second hand pleasure. The secret shared between Katherine and Samantha happens to most clinicians and as with these two it is an unpredictable communion. A sip from each other's cup - solemn, joyful and moving. It becomes a strong memory and refreshment that begs repeating.

COMMON DISEASES OCCUR COMMONLY

HERSHEY

"How'd you like to see a patient with Lyme disease?" The questioner was Ivo White, a surgeon friend of mine. He knows how to tickle my interest - I like to see patients with unusual illnesses and disorders. The rare disease, I'm convinced, holds much for the understanding of the common malady. The difficult diagnostic puzzle challenges your problem solving skills, keeps you thoughtful and is more fun than the best mystery novel.

To have a diagnosis is to have a hook on certainty - sometimes. A diagnosis is a label that presupposes a cause or at least familiarity. Someone else has seen the same thing and has put a name on it. The label can be prejudicial because the clinician sort of changes gears from, "What is wrong?" to "What should I do?" So it was that when C.P. Wainwright came into my office that I was prepared to deal with a case of Lyme disease.

"Hello Mr. Wainwright. How can I help you?" I asked.

"Got Lyme disease and I need a new doctor," he said.

"Had you been seeing Dr. White?" I asked.

"Oh, no. I was doing some work for Dr. White and asked him whom I should see. I'm a landscape architect and got to talking with Dr. White about my Lyme disease and how I needed a new doctor and he said I should see you."

"Well," I said, "tell me about your illness and how you think I can help you."

"It started about a year ago. I got some tick bites in my work - always seem to be getting tick bites. Then I got this rash and felt bad. Got a fever and sweats and felt awful. It lasted a couple of weeks off and on but I didn't see anybody about it. Then my sister said she saw this T.V. program about Lyme disease and she said that that was what I must have so I went to my family doctor and he started to treat me."

"What did your doctor do?" I asked.

"Well, he gave me some antibiotics and I felt much better," was the reply.

"Did he do some laboratory tests?"

"Oh yeah, he took some blood samples."

"Did he say what he thought was wrong with you?"

"Well yeah, he said I probably did have Lyme disease."

"How are you now?" I asked getting more curious about the reason for this visit.

"Ok now, but unless I take the antibiotics I get sick again and now my doctor says he's not going to give me any more because I should be all better. But I'm not. I think he just gave up on me!"

"Tell me more about your illness. Exactly what has been happening over the last year."?

"Well here, I brought you a whole bunch of info on Lyme disease," he said handing over a stack of torn magazine articles, photocopied flyers and a brochure from a Lyme organization. The latter, a group of patients and friends interested in the disease swapping notes, cautions and advice. This wasn't what I wanted. What I wanted was just a conversation about his illness. What he was telling me was that he had all of the preliminary material under control and now just wanted to get to the treatment part. He specifically pointed out to me that stubborn cases require intravenous antibiotics and wanted to know how soon we could get started since his supply of pills was soon to run out.

He began to grow impatient with my questioning. I sensed he was upset that I might not believe all he had been through, that I would not understand his weariness with feeling ill.

"OK, Mr. Wainwright. How about I take a look at you and then we talk about where to go from here?"

"What d'ya mean. You want to examine me? What for?"

"Well, it will be helpful to me if I know where we are now so that I can see what progress we make with treatment," I said.

"Well OK but the rash is gone and you aren't gonna find anything cause I been takin the antibiotic and now I feel good," he said with resignation.

He was right - almost. The examination was really quite normal except that following the rectal examination there was a very faint blush of blue on the Hemoccult card. Perhaps I disturbed a fissure or hemorrhoid - perhaps not. I told him about the exam including the trace of blood in his stool and asked about symptoms of ulcer disease, which he denied.

"How about your bowels, Mr. Wainwright?"

"Well they haven't been too good cause of all the antibiotics. I tend to constipation and have to take lots of laxatives to keep em moving," he said.

"Ever see any blood in you bowel movements?"

"Yeah, but my doc said I had hemorrhoids."

"Well, I didn't see any but perhaps you have some internal hemorrhoids."

"Doc," he said now getting quite upset, "it's not my bowels I came to see you about. I don't want to miss any more work and I'm really tired of feeling bad and taking pills!"

Deal time, I thought. Time to make a deal. I've been here before. How do you get the job done and keep everyone happy. The art of negotiating can be as important in the doctor's office as in the corporate boardroom.

"Okay, Mr. Wainwright. Here's what I suggest we do. Let me run a few blood tests on you today." The scowl on his face hastens me to add, "and I'll give you some more antibiotics till I see you next week. In the meantime, I want to call your doctor and find out the results of his tests so we can put this all together and find out how to get you over this problem. How's that sound?" His sigh was my only clue that he'd go along with this plan. I also got him to agree to take a few stool test cards along and bring them back the next week.

There were many phone calls over that week. I talked with his doctor and indeed he had a slightly elevated antibody titer to the Lyme spirochete about nine months earlier but it had not been repeated. I called our laboratory to find that his test was now negative. His sisters both called me with independent advice about how to treat CP's Lyme disease. They both called him CP and had both decided that he had the disease. His wife called to know if I thought it would be covered under Worker's compensation and wasn't there some kind of legislation to control this disease. All three indicated that it was all right for CP to see me but they also knew of some experts in Lyme disease and didn't I think maybe he should see them. Frankly, I was beginning to think that was a pretty good idea.

C.P. came back and reported that he was feeling well. Wasn't I satisfied now he wondered and couldn't we get on with the important business at hand and start the intravenous antibiotics?

The problem was, all of the stool cards he brought back showed blood.

Let's see now, Lyme disease without any antibody titer and with blood in the stool. Rare manifestations of a rare disease make clinicians nervous. In this case, the family now shared a comfort in the Lyme disease cocoon. Once a diagnosis and a patient are hooked together it can be hard to twist them apart. No one likes to admit they were wrong.

"C.P, you still have blood in your stool. I would like take a look at your lower bowel with an instrument and see if you have some hemorrhoids or something else causing the bleeding."

"You mean you want to stick one of those tubes up my behind don't you?" he asked with anger. "No way doc. My buddy had one of those and said it was awful. Can't you do an x-ray or something?"

Deal time again. "OK, C.P. we can do an x-ray of your colon. It's called a barium enema."

Exasperated, C.P. agreed just as long as we could then "get on with it!"

The x-ray showed a large apple core lesion. It was a typical picture of cancer of the colon. In addition there was a small tract of barium that filled an adjacent abscess. Common diseases occur commonly. C.P.'s illness now made sense. The antibiotics concealed the presence of the pus pocket and made him feel well enough to tolerate the inexorable growth of the tumor. Sooner or later of course he would have obstructed his colon and would have shown the weight loss and spread to his liver for which this cancer is well known. The question now was how much later were we? At least nine months of symptoms had passed. Nine months of chances for cells to break free from the tumor slip through his blood stream and nest in far away organs.

Surgery was arranged after passing a cup of chagrin all around. There was a general truce in the conversation and a quiet time till the day of surgery. The surgery was difficult since the abscess had caused dense adhesions around the area of the tumor. It was removed along with a generous wedge of the mesentery and as many lymph nodes as could be dissected along the root of the mesentery and the aorta.

Fools have great luck and so it was that we were told two days later by the pathology department that all of the lymph nodes were free of disease and that the tumor seemed to be contained. The abscess was not a tumor abscess but an adjacent diverticular abscess. The nub was that C.P. had probably been cured of his disease.

I rejoiced with the family. It's a thrill to see the enthusiasms for the routine come upon those who have had a close call. It's like someone turned up the intensity of the lights. Small things are noticed and relished, food tastes better, courtesies are extended easily, the newspaper is more interesting, and talk is more refreshing. My vicarious participation was dulled just a bit on the day of discharge. Mrs. Wainwright asked, "Doctor, how soon can we start on the antibiotics for his Lyme Disease?"

THE PURPOSE OF MEDICINE

MISCELLANY

A notion of the purpose of medicine, to be helpful, should be both encompassing and delimiting. It aught define those things that doctors do as distinct from what others do. To say that the purpose of medicine is to help the sick (a common assertion) is neither comprehensive nor specific. Medical examiners and public health physicians do not care for the sick. Clergy and others care for the sick and are not doctors. To get closer to a helpful description of the purpose of medicine inevitably leads to the use of some common words - words that also beg for clarity. The reason we might want to explore these words is more than to dispel sophistry. I thought we might be able to drive to a clearer understanding of the purpose of medicine since that, for the most part, is our business.

I propose that we discuss some definitions in medicine for our Friday lunch. These are common terms, which because of their commonness are taken as standards. These terms have a sense of intuitive identification but lead to great confusion when one attempts precise definition.

Attached are excerpts from a number of blind elephant grabbers to stimulate your thoughts.

Finally, the last page is just for fun. It is a list of things that doctors are called upon to tend to (with a couple of exceptions). Can we decide on the purpose of medicine as activities, which doctors do?

DEFINITION OF HEALTH
"A STATE OF COMPLETE PHYSICAL, MENTAL AND SOCIAL WELL-BEING, AND NOT MERELY THE ABSENCE OF DISEASE OR INFIRMITY."
FROM: BASIC DOCUMENTS, 26TH EDITION, WHO, GENEVA, 1976

IS ANYBODY HEALTHY?

1. THE REFERENCE CLASS IS A NATURAL CLASS OF OR-
GANISMS OF UNIFORM FUNCTIONAL DESIGN; SPECIFICAL-
LY, AN AGE GROUP OF A SEX OF A SPECIES.

2. A NORMAL FUNCTION OF A PART OR PROCESS WITH-
IN MEMBERS OF THE REFERNCE CLASS IS A STATISTICALLY
TYPICAL CONTRIBUTION TO THEIR INDIVIDUAL SURVIVAL
AND REPRODUCTION.

3. HEALTH IN A MEMBER OF THE REFERENCE CLASS IS
NORMAL FUNCTIONAL ABILITY; THE READINESS OF EACH
PART TO PERFORM ALL ITS NORMAL FUNCTIONS ON TYPI-
CAL OCCASIONS WITH AT LEAST TYPICAL EFFICIENCY.
HEALTH IS THE ABSENCE OF DISEASE
FROM: BOORSE C: HEATLH AS A THEORETICAL CON-
CEPT.
PHILOS SCI 1977;44:542-573

LOTS OF ROOM FOR NORMATIVES AND VALUES

A DISEASE IS A STATE OF THE HUMAN ORGANISM THAT
ACTUALLY OR POTENTIALLY DISADVANTAGES A PERSON
FOR SURVIVAL, REPRODUCTION OR FULL ENJOYMENT OF
LIFE (CHARACTERISTIC FOR AGE) OTHER THAN BY SOLE
REASON OF SOCIAL CIRCUMSTANCE OR BY TEMPORARY
AND REVERSIBLE ENVIRONMENTAL CHANGE.
FROM: EMSON HE, HEALTH, DISEASE AND ILLNESS: MAT-
TERS FOR DEFINITION. CAN MED ASSOC J 1987;136:811-813

JOHN W. BURNSIDE, M.D.

BIOMEDICAL DISEASE IS DEMONSTRABLE PATHOPHYSI-OLOGY OR PATHOCHEMISTRY AND IS DIAGNOSED BY THE DEMONSTRATION OF PATHOLOGIC FEATURES. DISEASE IS A MATTER OF PHYSICS AND CHEMISTRY. ILLNESSES ARE THE OPPOSITE OF HEALTH AND ARE SUBJECTIVELY EXPE-RIENCED PHENOMENA.

ILLNESS IS EXPERIENCE AND ONLY DISEASE CAN BE IN-VESTIGATED BY THE METHODS OF BIOMEDICINE BECAUSE THE STUDY OF ILLNESS DEPENDS DIRECTLY ON PHENOM-ENOLOGIC ANALYSIS OF EXPERIENCED SUFFERING.

ONE CAN BE SERIOUSLY DISEASED WITHOUT BEING ILL AND ONE CAN BE SERIOUSLY ILL WITHOUT BEING DISEASED.

FROM: JENNINGS D: THE CONFUSION BETWEEN DISEASE AND ILLNESS IN CLINICAL MEDICINE. CAN MED ASSOC J 1986;135:865-870

IFIND THIS DISTINCTION HELPFUL - HOW ABOUT YOU?

DISEASE MAY BE VIEWED AS A BIOLOGIC EVENT, CHAR-ACTERIZED BY ANATOMIC, PHYSIOLOGIC OR BIOCHEMICAL CHANGES, OR BY SOME MIXTURE OF THESE. IT IS A DISRUP-TION IN THE STRUCTURE AND OR FUNCTION OF A BODY PART OR SYSTEM. IT MAY BE DUE TO A VARIETY OF CAUSES, MAY PERSIST, ADVANCE OR REGRESS THROUGH A VARIETY OF MECHANISMS, AND MAY OR MAY NOT BE CLINICALLY APPARENT.

ILLNESS, ON THE OTHER HAND, IS NOT A BIOLOG-IC BUT A HUMAN EVENT. IT CONSISTS OF AN ARRAY OF DISCOMFORTS AND PSYCHOSOCIAL DISLOCATIONS RE-SULTING FROM INTERACTION OF A PERSON WITH THE

ENVIRONMENT. BARONDESS JA. DISEASE AND ILLNESS - A CRUCIAL DISTINCTION. AM J MED 1979;66:375-6

...CHOOSING TO CALL A SET OF PHENOMENA A DISEASE INVOLVES A COMMITMENT TO MEDICAL INTERVENTION

...WHAT COUNTS AS HEALTH AND DISEASE FOR HUMANS DEPENDS UPON VERY COMPLEX JUDGEMENTS CONCERNING SUFFERING, THE GOALS PROPER TO HUMANS, AND THE FORM OR APPEARANCE PROPER TO HUMANS.
ENGLEHARDT HT, THE CONCEPTS OF HEALTH AND DISEASE. IN EVALUATION AND EXPLANATION IN THE BIO-MEDICAL SCIENCES. ED BY ENGLEHARDT, SPICKER AND DORDRECHT: REIDEL, 1975

THIS HAS THE RING OF TRUTH - IS IT A GOOD THING?

"CONCENTRATION ON THE TECHNICAL ASPECTS OF CARE HAS DIVERTED US FROM THE PATIENT'S INNER WORLD, AN ASPECT OF ILLLNESS THE (SCIENTIFIC) METHOD DOES NOT ROUTINELY FORCE ON OUR ATTENTION"
MCWHINNEY IR, ARE WE ON THE BRINK OF A MA-JOR TRANSFORMATION OF CLINICAL METHOD? CMAJ 1986;135:873-878

MEDICINE IS A NARROW DISCIPLINE. IT DOES NOT PRO-MOTE THE REALIZATION OF HAPPINESS, INNER TRANQUIL-ITY, MORAL NOBILITY, GOOD CITIZENSHIP. BUT IT CAN BRING TO BEAR AN INCREASINGLY POWERFUL CONCEPTUAL

SYSTEM FOR THE MITIGATION OF HUMAN SUFFERING ROOT-
ED IN BIOMEDICAL DISTURBANCES.

A CONCERN FOR HUMAN LIFE IS THERFORE NOT IPSO
FACTO A MEDICAL CONCERN

ITS (MEDICINE'S) GOALS MAY BE DEFINED AS THE RE-
LIEF OF PAIN, THE PREVENTION OF DISABILITY, AND THE
POSTPONEMENT OF DEATH BY THE APPLICATION OF THE
THEORETICAL KNOWLEDGE INCORPORATED IN MEDICAL
SCIENCE TO INDIVIDUAL PATIENTS.

...THE MEDICALIZATION OF HUMAN EXPERIENCE LEADS
TO...FRUSTRATION AND DISILLUSIONMENT WHEN MEDICAL
INTERVENTION FAILS TO EVENTUATE IN TRANQUILITY,
QUIESCENCE, AND HAPPINESS.
SELDIN DW. PRESIDENTIAL ADDRESS. THE BOUNDAR-
IES OF MEDICINE. TRANS ASSOC AM PHYSICIANS 1981;94:
LXXV-LXXXVI

OUR OWN DON SELDIN WOULD FROM THIS VIEW,
EXCLUDE MUCH OF WHAT DOCTORS DO AS INAPPROPRIATE
TO THE PRACTICE OF MEDICINE.

"WHAT I WOULD CLAIM...IS THAT THE TECHNICAL
EXPERTISE OF THE DOCTOR/ SCIENTIST IS NEITHER
SUFFICIENT NOR NECESSARY FOR THE ATTRIBUTION OF
'DISEASE' AND THAT THIS ATTRIBUTION IS BASED ON
CONVENTIONAL VALUES" BIRCH J. A MSICONCEPTION
CONCERNING THE MEANING OF 'DISEASE'. BRIT J MED
PSYCH 1979;52:367-75

'...ANY DEFINITION OF DISEASE WHICH BOILS DOWN TO "WHAT PEOPLE COMPLAIN OF" OR "WHAT DOCTORS TREAT", OR SOME COMBINATION OF THE TWO...IS FREE TO EXPAND OR CONTRACT WITH CHANGES IN SOCIAL ATTITUDES AND THERAPEUTIC OPTIMISM AND IS AT THE MERCY OF IDIOSYNCRATIC DECISIONS BY DOCTOR OR PATIENTS."

KENDALL RE, THE CONCEPT OF DISEASE AND ITS IMPLICATIONS FOR PSYCHIATRY. BRIT J PSYCH 1975; 127:305-315

THE INCLUSION OR EXCLUSION OF VALUES AND NORMATIVE SOCIAL DIMENSIONS JOINS MANY AUTHORS PROCLAMATIONS. NOTICE THE NEXT TWO EXCERPTS.

THE HALLMARK OF DISEASE IS THERAPEUTIC CONCERN BY AN INDIVIDUAL OR BY OTHERS IN THE FACE OF SOME ABNORMAL MANIFESTATION. THERE ARE, FOR EXAMPLE, SOCIAL MISFITS AND EMOTIONALLY UNSTABLE PERSONS WHO CAN AROUSE EITHER THERAPEUTIC OR PUNITIVE CONCERN IN THOSE AROUND THEM. IT IS ONLY WHEN THE THERAPEUTIC CONCERN GAINS THE UPPER HAND, AT LEAST TEMPORARILY,

THAT SUCH PERSONS ARE CONSIDERED BELONGING TO THE CLASS OF PATIENTS.

KRAUPL-TAYLOR F. A LOGICAL ANALYSIS OF THE MEDICO-PSYCHOLOGICAL CONCEPT OF DISEASE. PSYCH MED 1971;1:356-364

JOHN W. BURNSIDE, M.D.

"WHILE PROFESSIONALS HAVE A MAJOR VOICE IN INFLUENCING THE JUDGMENT OF SOCIETY, IT IS THE COLLECTIVE JUDGMENT OF THE LARGER SOCIAL GROUP THAT DETERMINES WHETHER ITS MEMBERS ARE TO BE VIEWED AS SICK OR CRIMINAL, ECCENTRIC OR IMMORAL"
GREGORY, I. FUNDAMENTALS OF PSYCHIATRY. 1968 W.B. SAUNDERS, PHILADELPHIA

SINCE THE HUMAN BODY (UNLIKE SOCIAL INSTITUTIONS) HAS CHANGED RELATIVELY LITTLE OVER MILLENIA, THE FUNCTIONAL NORMS OF SOMATIC MEDICINE ARE RELATIVELY CONSERVATIVE (UNLIKE THE NORMS OF LAW). BUT SINCE, UNDERSTANDABLY ENOUGH, MEDICINE HAS EXPANDED ITS PURVIEW TO INCLUDE THE CONCERNS OF MENTAL HEALTH AND MENTAL ILLNESS, AND SINCE MEDICINE IN GENERAL MUST SUBSERVE, HOWEVER CONSERVATIVELY,

THE DETERMINATE IDEOLOGY AND ULTERIOR GOALS OF GIVEN SOCIETIES, THE ACTUAL CONCEPTION OF DISEASES CANNOT BUT REFLECT THE STATE OF THE TECHNOLOGY, THE SOCIAL EXPECTATIONS, THE DIVISION OF LABOR, AND THE ENVIRONMENTAL CONDITION OF THOSE POPULATIONS.

IN A SENSE, THEREFORE, MEDICINE IS IDEOLOGY RESTRICTED BY OUR SENSE OF THE MINIMAL REQUIREMENTS OF THE FUNCTIONAL INTEGRITY OF THE BODY AND MIND (HEALTH) ENABLING (PRUDENTIALLY) THE CHARACTERISTIC ACTIVITIES AND INTERESTS OF THE RACE TO BE PURSUED. AND DISEASE IS WHATEVER IS JUDGED TO DISORDER OR TO CAUSE TO DISORDER, IN THE RELEVANT WAY, THE MINIMAL INTEGRITY OF BODY AND MIND RELATIVE TO

PRUDENTIAL FUNCTIONS. MARGOLIS J. THE CONCEPT OF DISEASE. J MED AND PHIL. 1976;1:238-255

THESE NORMATIVE CONCEPTS ARE NOWHERE OF GREATER CONCERN THAN IN PSYCHIATRY.

ONE NEED ONLY GLANCE AT THE DIAGNOSTIC MANUAL OF THE AMERICAN PSYCHIATRIC ASSOCIATION TO LEARN WHAT AN ELASTIC CONCEPT MENTAL ILLNESS IS.

IT RANGES FROM THE MASSIVE FUNCTIONAL INHI-BITION CHARACTERISTIC OF ONE FORM OF CATATONIC SCHIZOPHRENIA TO THOSE SEEMINGLY SLIGHT ABERRAN-CIES ASSOCIATED WITH AN UNSTABLE PERSONALITY, BUT WHICH ARE SO CLOSE TO CONDUCT IN WHICH WE ALL EN-GAGE AS TO DEFINE THE ENTIRE CONTINUUM INVOLVED... AND, BECAUSE OF THE UNAVOIDABLY AMBIGUOUS

GENERALITIES IN WHICH THE AMERICAN PSYCHIATRIC ASSOCIATION DESCRIBES ITS DIAGNOSTIC CATEGORIES, THE DIAGNOSTICIAN HAS THE ABILITY TO SHOEHORN INTO THE MENTALLY DISEASED CLASS ALMOST ANY PERSON HE WISHES, FOR WHATEVER REASON, TO PUT THERE.

LIVERMORE JM ET.AL. ON THE JUSTIFICATIONS FOR CIVIL COMMITMENT. UNIV. PENN LAW REVIEW 1968;117:75-96

"IT WILL BE RECALLED THAT CRITICAL THEORY IN PSYCHIATRY HAS TENDED TO POSTULATE A FUNDAMENTAL SEPARATION BETWEEN MENTAL ILLNESSES AND THE GENERAL RUN OF HUMAN AILMENTS: THE FORMER ARE

THE EXPRESSION OF SOCIAL NORMS, THE LATTER PROCEED FROM ASCERTAINABLE BODILY STATES WHICH HAVE AN "OBJECTIVE" EXISTENCE WITHIN THE INDIVIDUAL."

SEDGWICK OBJECTS TO THIS DISTINCTION.

THE MEDICAL ENTERPRISE IS FROM ITS INCEPTION VALUE-LOADED: IT IS NOT SIMPLY AN APPLIED BIOLOGY, BUT BIOLOGY APPLIED IN ACCORDANCE WITH THE DICTATES OF SOCIAL INTEREST.

ALL SICKNESS IS ESSENTIALLY DEVIANCY.

ALL ILLNESS, WHETHER CONCEIVED IN LOCALIZED BODILY

TERMS OR WITHIN A LARGER VIEW OF HUMAN FUNC-TIONING, EXPRESSES BOTH A LARGER VIEW OF HUMAN FUNCTIONING, EXPRESSES BOTH A SOCIAL VALUE- JUDG-MENT (CONTRASTING A PERSON'S CONDITION WITH CER-TAIN UNDERSTOOD AND ACCEPTED NORMS) AND AN ATTEMPT AT EXPLANATION (WITH A VIEW TO CONTROL-LING THE DISVALUED CONDITION).

SEDGWICK P. ILLNESS - MENTAL AND OTHERWISE IN PSCYHO POLITICS 1982 HARPER AND ROW

(THANKS TO JOHN SADLER FOR THIS ONE)

PERHAPS THE ROLE OF MEDICINE IS TO TEND TO "SICK" PEOPLE

"...THE SICK ROLE: (1) THE SICK PERSON IS EXEMPTED FROM THOSE SOCIAL RESPONSIBILITIES IMPEDED BY HIS OR HER ILLNESS OR DEFORMITY;(2) THE STATE OF AFFAIRS IS NOT ONE DEPENDING IMMEDIATELY UPON THE WILL OF

THE SICK INDIVIDUAL (E.G. IT CANNOT BE SIMPLY WILLED AWAY, AS IN THE CASE OF MALINGERING); (3) THE ILL OR SICK PERSON IS EXPECTED TO COOPERATE IN GETTING WELL OR AT LEAST STAYING AS WELL AS POSSIBLE; AND (4) THE ILL OR SICK PERSON IS EXPECTED TO SEEK OUT APPROPRIATE "MEDICAL TREATMENT". THE SICK ROLE DESCRIBES CERTAIN PATTERNS OF BEHAVIOR ASSOCIATED WITH STATES OF ILLNESS AS WELL AS SOME STATES OF DEFORMITY AND EXPANDS THE MEANING OF BEING ILL BY GIVING IT A SOCIAL DIMENSION." ENGLEHARDT HT, IDEOLOGY AND ETIOLOGY. J.MED AND PHIL. 1976;1;256-268

CLOUSER, FRUSTRATED WITH THE ATTEMPTS AT DEFI-NITION OF HEALTH AND DISEASE SUGGESTS THAT THE TERM "MALADY" HAS MUCH TO BE SAID FOR IT IN OUR DELIBERATIONS

THE TERM "MALADY" THOUGH MORE GENERAL THAN THE COMMONLY USED RELATED TERMS, IS NEVERTHELESS EXPLICIT, PRECISE AND USABLE. A PERSON HAS A MALADY IF AN ONLY IF HE HAS A CONDITION, OTHER THAN HIS RATIO-NAL BELIEFS AND DESIRES, SUCH THAT HE IS SUFFERING, OR AT INCREASED RISK OF SUFFERING, AN EVIL (DEATH, PAIN, DISABILITY, LOSS OF FREEDOM OR OPPORTUNITY, OR LOSS OF PLEASURE) IN THE ABSENCE OF A DISTINCT SUS-TAINING CAUSE.

CLOUSER KD, CULVER CM, GERT B. MALADY: A NEW TREATMENT OF DISEASE. HASTINGS CENTER REPORT 1981;11:29-37

AFTER ALL THIS I'M WEAK, TIRED, AND DIZZY. I WONDER IF I'M SICK. TRY ATTACHING A DESCRIPTOR(S) TO THE FOLLOWING:

DISEASE, ILLNESS, MALADY, DEVIANCY, PROCESS, MOR-BUS, INJURY, INFIRMITY, DISORDER, ILLTH OR ANYTHING ELSE, WHICH FITS

1. FRACTURED ARM
2. NON EXPRESSED CHROMOSOMAL TRANSLOCATION
3. TEENAGE PREGNANCY
4. BALDNESS
5. DEATH
6. DEPRESSION
7. HYPERCHOLESTEROLEMIA
8. SMOKING
9. CYCLE RIDING WITHOUT A HELMET
10. HOMOSEXUALITY
11. OLD AGE
12. ATHEROSCLEROSIS IN A CHILD/ADULT/OCTOGENARIAN
13. IQ OF 70
14. FERTILITY
15. CELIBACY
16. DRAPETOMANIA*
17. UGLINESS
18. PAIN OF A PROPER HUMAN FUCNTION (TEETHING, CHILDBIRTH}
19. COMA

*DRAPETOMANIA"
– THE UNEXPLAINED DESIRE OF SLAVES TO RUN AWAY.

INTERFERENCE

DALLAS

Metropolitan Friday evenings are filled with people things. Streets, theaters, restaurants and emergency rooms share the exuberance of "no work tomorrow."

The emergency room of the Massachusetts General Hospital was almost always busy but especially so on Friday nights. The local knife and gun club used us as a dressing room and the stubborn coughs, aches and pains finally became too much and demanded attention. Even coronary and cerebral arteries seemed to relish mischief on Friday nights.

During residency training, you spend time in the emergency room each year of your training. With each year of seniority, the task assigned differs until the most senior year when you are assigned the duty of triage officer. You make very quick assessments of patients at the front desk to find the nature of the problem and the degree of urgency and so direct patients, other residents and staff. At the time, it appeared to be a demotion to be moved from the action rooms to traffic duty. Now, I know that to be the most important task in emergency medicine. You have to make the most difficult diagnosis in that role. You have to be able to diagnose "sick". When mistakes are made in emergency medicine, they can be most commonly traced to the failure to diagnose "sick" when a patient is, or to the diagnosis of "sick" when the patient is not.

This particular Friday night was like others - busy. All of the exam rooms were occupied, the waiting room filled with the walking wounded or sick at heart. Everyone was on a short string, barely civil and wary of his or her own priorities. Clerks minded their mentors by securing the right paper work. If the family doesn't speak English, just shout louder. Residents worked the "iron door" policy - don't admit unless absolutely necessary since an admission will only get you grief from the beleaguered team on the ward. X-ray was backed up - why hurry, we're paid by the hour not the piece. There was no degree of urgency, which hadn't been seen before, and too much sense that it really didn't make a whole lot of difference. Not a very humane place. Far from the high drama portrayed on TV.

A pod of five or six patients had just been dealt with when an ambulance driver asked to transfer a waiting patient to one of our litters so they could be on their way. All of the regular ambulance crews knew to do this. Making them return later because the patient was not admitted taught them that an ambulance ride was not diagnostic of "sick". So, they would wait for the triage before scurrying away.

There was a small lump on the litter. A blanket was tucked around the lump and because it was cold, there was a towel around the patient's head. Peeling off the layers, I found an ancient woman. She didn't move. She was curled in a fetal position. Her waxy skin was pulled taught over a tiny boned frame. She had thin silvery hair, a blank stare and a claw hand of an old stroke. Slipping a cold stethoscope under a fleshless breast, I asked what was the matter not expecting a reply.

Her good hand slipped out from under her body and grasped my wrist with strength. Her eyes rolled around to fix on mine and in a surprisingly clear voice she said, "Sonny, I've come here to die and I'll brook no interference on your part!"

I remember to this day my sense of astonishment and shame. Dignity slapped my hand. The shape of the body rarely portrays the shape of the mind. Here was the ultimate in patient autonomy.

She was admitted without a specific diagnosis although I was sure she was "sick". She died three days later. We did try to interfere and she had none of it. Since then other patients have announced their impending death to me and I take it very very seriously. Is it premonition or planning?

KINGS QUEENS AND ROOKERIES

DALLAS

Since coming to Dallas, I have an office with a view. My eleventh floor corner office looks over the plaza of the campus. A lovely place of brick, planters, trellises and small benches for respite. Across from the plaza is the Egret rookery, a protected copse of trees where year after year Egrets take up residence, breed, and brood and raise their young. They arrive suddenly and depart the same way. The rookery means different things to different people. Students like the patch of green and many like the notion of a safe haven for something wild and natural within the city. Others look longingly at this space of perhaps three acres and see the solution to the constant need for new offices and laboratories.

Within the rookery is a common grave. It's a flat concrete pad with a handsome non-denominational marker. The pad has a lid through which new remains can be constantly added to the old. What goes through the grate are the powders and bone shards from the crematorium - our crematorium. The stack of the crematorium can also be seen from my window between the plaza and the rookery. It is often in use, I can tell by the shimmering distortion of the view beyond and the occasional puffs of black or white smoke. The final remains of the bodies and body parts used for education and research can be seen from my window - gases up and powder down through the grate.

The King and Queen of Sweden came to Dallas. They came to the medical school to visit and acknowledge the three Noble laureates on our campus. The plaza was beautiful and festive with flowers, a red carpet and a nervous reception committee. The royal couple was gracious visitors as the dignitaries greeted them. The Queen received a special bouquet from Stormy Jones a young girl who was the first heart and liver transplant patient in the world. She was there because of her significance in the discovery of special cholesterol receptors by Michael Brown and Joseph Goldstein, two of the laureates.

We are a large campus with more than 4,000 who work and study here. Communications are sometimes difficult and there was a failure to distribute all of the proper protocol for visiting royalty.

Somehow the part that says "don't use the crematorium when the King and Queen are on campus", failed to reach the proper operator.

Out of the corner of my eye, I saw the first belch of smoke. Over the next twenty minutes there was a faint blush of smoke and shimmering.

I'm sure not many people noticed the smoke or even the faint sweet acrid smell. I did see the royal nose twitch - I'm sure I did. A few others glanced at each other with a quick knowing arch of brows.

What to make of all of this I'm not sure. Was this a reminder of the final common pathway amidst this celebration of science, life and a sunny day? Or, was it just a funny thing that happened? As I said, I'm not sure what to make of it. I don't really think of such things very often. My clinical and educational work is with the living. Death comes after me.

MEDICINE ON A GRAND SCALE

BOSTON

My brother Dan is smarter than me. He is a veterinarian. He is the oldest and I am the youngest of four brothers. Dan had always wanted to be a veterinarian just as I had always wanted to be a physician. His enthusiasm for his dream affected me and he taught me about grit. Wanting something hard was not enough you had to twist the want into tolerance for fatigue, nonsense and time.

Dan applied early for veterinary school but was not admitted until shortly before classes began. He worried for months and also applied to medical school to which he was readily admitted. When it appeared that the vet school was not going to admit him he accepted the invitation from Jefferson Medical School and was beginning to adjust to the notion of people over cows when he finally got the news that the University of Pennsylvania Veterinary School would give him a chance. He lived at home to save money and commuted daily to Philadelphia developing a routine of flagellant discipline. I was still in high school and watched this pilgrimage with fascination. He was usually out of the house before I got up, came home for a late supper (we waited for him) and went immediately to his room to study. His bedroom was large enough for a recliner and the recliner was large enough for Dan - he's a big fellow. With a floor lamp behind his left shoulder and a board across the arms of the recliner, he would read and write forever. I could come into the room but could only rarely talk. I delighted in flipping the pages of his enormous books with particular pleasure in Gray's Anatomy, which became the first chapter in the mystery I am still reading. Once in a great while, we would bullshit and he would regale me with some outrageous tale of an inept classmate or curious animal or hardass professor.

Everything about Dan is grand and big. He eats with real gusto, his laughter is rich and full, he throws spadefuls in the garden with force and his anger is best avoided. It was no surprise then that he chose a practice involving large animals. He had little tolerance for the dog and cat trade. Not that he didn't like the little creatures; it was that he didn't like their owners. Farmers, barns, tractors, cows, horses and pigs - these were important things, livelihood things, earthy things. He began practice in a group in Buck's County in Quakertown and quickly became a regular sight on the back roads with his specially loaded pick up truck clouding from one farm to another. Big tools, big pills and big animals.

While he was establishing himself as that 'young vet', I was struggling through medical school and residency. When I graduated from medical school he suggested, only half in jest that we go into practice together. "We can put up a big sign - Burnside and Burnside - Man or Beast!" he said. I still think of that notion from time to time especially when his brand of silent medicine seems particularly sweet.

How nice, I sometimes think, to just go ahead and do what is right and not have to travel the conversation road, fill out the forms, make the phone calls, alert the clerks and ask Mother may I. Just me and a big sick cow - wow! This, of course, is not the case, as any vet will tell you. In fact, I have been with Dan when the conversation takes a long time. It sometimes becomes a disturbing conversation, foreign to my brand of medicine.

"Well, Les. She's got nails!"
"Ach, Doc. You mean you gotta cut her?"
"Either that or she goes to the baloney maker, Les." "How much to fix her, Doc?"

"About $600 Les and then she'll be off her milk till next freshening."

"Well, let me see, she gives about 600 pounds...."
And so the conversation and computation goes - medical economics.

Still it is medicine on a grand scale and I took what few opportunities I could to make rounds with Dan. The standard unit of this part of the agricultural world is 200 acres under till and about 40 milk cows. This unit is worked by the basic family unit of farmer, working wife, two children and a sometimes hand.

The drill I came to know consisted of driving into the yard with a flourish, beep the horn and go forthwith into the barn. At first, I didn't understand this apparent rudeness of not waiting to be led in but later I realized that the call was business and that the business was in the barn and you'd better get to the business. Also, I suspect, there was a fun game involved which was to stroll into the barn of forty cattle and with a quick glance go unerringly to the stanchion bordering the sick beast. I don't yet know how this is done. The cows all looked pretty much the same to me, the manure seemed the same and the farmer never tied a ribbon to the sick one. The only clue I ever tumbled to was that occasionally the fodder trough in front of the sick one still had hay or grain in it.

On one occasion a scratchy call came over the radio to visit a farmer who had a cow with "milk fever." Dan explained that this was neither a fever nor did it have much to do with milk. Cows he taught me don't get a lot of calcium in their diet and when called on to nourish a calf in the womb much of their calcium reserve is used up.

After calving, this calcium deficiency is sometimes severe enough to give the beast great trouble and it constituted a veterinary emergency.

This time, instead of going to the barnyard we cruised slowly along the pasture fence line until Dan spotted the cow lying on her side in the sun. Others were about her chewing cud unaware of their stricken sister. This time I felt my diagnosis was certain. This cow was dead.

It was clear to me. She was motionless, four legs stretched out straight and there were flies walking over her glazed eyes. Why then were we hauling boxes and bottles over the field around the pies?

"Have her up in a minute," Dan said.

"No way brother. Call the dead animal man."

"Watch. This is my favorite."

He produced a needle about the size of a #2 Eberhard pencil, slammed it into the neck of the beast producing a small fountain of blood. Then attaching what looked to be a small garden hose he glugged in two liters of a 50% calcium solution. Two liters! 50% calcium! If this cow wasn't dead this surely was the euthanizing solution, I thought. I knew what milligrams and milliliters of calcium could do to a human and this dose gave me palpitations.

Before the solution was completely delivered the cow began to tremble all over, her legs flailed in a trot against the air, she had a massive bowel movement and stood up! The eye glaze disappeared and before Dan could stow all of his equipment she began to graze. Lazarus.

"Wow!" was my comment.

"No big deal," said Dan but I could tell from his sly grin that he was pleased to once again astonish his little brother.

Lynda, my wife, was a frequent audience to my tales of brother Dan. She too seemed fascinated by these grand stories and frequently expressed the desire to see it herself.

"Particularly a calving," she would say to both of us. We visited one weekend having driven to Quakertown from Boston to get away from residency for a little bit and to share our pleasure at Lynda's increasing gravid condition - about 5 months pregnant with our first son. While we were enjoying coffee and conversation after supper the call came for Dan to attend a difficult calving. "Yes, of course I want to go," and "No, it won't bother me in the least," were her rapid-fire responses.

Lynda is no stranger to blood and gore. She has worked as a pediatric nurse and in a surgical recovery room and the squeems of that atmosphere had long been suppressed. This, however, was a somewhat different atmosphere. There are few analogies between a barn and a recovery room. Not only that but Lynda had never been in a barn! This fact was even unknown to me until we walked into the barn and her first query had to do with animal's being "barn trained" as she looked with disdain at the manure trough. She looked about as if to find the linen carts, surgical drapes and masks.

There was a chill in the evening air but in the barn there was the warmth of the large bodies and the pleasant smell of animals and straw. A string of bare light bulbs along the barn dropped cones of light along the way. This time I had no trouble identifying the patient. She was spread legged, her back was arched and she was bawling loud and long. Protruding from her vagina were two hoofs and feet and leaning across her back was a weary farmer stripped to the waist shiny with sweat.

"Sorry Doc, but she's really got one crosswise. I just can't budge her," said the farmer.

"Let's have a look," Dan said. He slipped his coveralls off his shoulders and tied the arms around his waist. He slid his hand, then wrist, then forearm and a lot of his upper arm into the cow's womb. It was like reaching for the broom handle stuck way back between the refrigerator and the wall. Lynda watched this disappearing act and some of her color went with Dan's arm.

"We gotta start over," said Dan withdrawing his arm only to now take both small hooves and push them back into the womb with repeated shoves like rocking a car stuck in the snow. With a slurp, they disappeared.

Immediately the cow tried to reverse things again with renewed bellowing and grunting.

"Now we get the other end," said Dan flipping open his Sear's Mastercraftsman toolbox and withdrawing two stainless steel link chains with rings at the ends. One at a time these were threaded through and around parts of the calf we could not see and that Dan could only feel.

Now with two lengths of chain dangling he attached rope hawsers to each, smiled and beckoned the farmer and me to a tug of war. Lynda's color thermometer dropped a few more degrees. We backed up to get some purchase from the stanchion across the isle and leaned to the task. I feared for the awful pressure we were developing. Surely everything will rent and tear. Finally with a great slopping plud the calf was delivered, the bellowing stopped and the cow looked back at her newborn. Mother and child were fine. Mother to be was not so sure. Dan was pleased. There's not often an amphitheater to his surgery.

"Time to sterilize the equipment," he said. A stainless steel bucket with steaming hot water, almost a fixture in milk barns, was produced. Squatting over the bucket, he squirted in a generous dollop of "Mr. Clean" and began running the chains up and down through the liquid. Cocking his head to the side with a grin looking at Lynda he said, "Would you like my card?"

PASSING STONES

HERSHEY

S ome doctors practice too long. Some realize it but don't act while others miss the signals as do their colleagues and friends. I learned that suggesting retirement to a colleague can be as therapeutic as a writing a prescription.

Some time ago, I had such a doctor as a patient. He had sent me a few patients for consultation so I knew who he was from our phone conversations. The patients that he sent were not particularly difficult diagnostic problems and I later felt that they had been his advance guard to test the waters. They had in common an intense loyalty to this doctor, and spent much of their visits telling me that he was a fine man and had taken care of them for years.

His first visit required several phone conversations between our office secretaries to check, change and double check appointment times. Yes, we would be certain to allot enough time. Yes, it would be fine if the doctor told me himself the nature of the visit and no, we wouldn't do any testing prior to his seeing me. Thank you very much.

During that first visit, he did a lot of bluster and posturing. It seemed he wished to portray that he was very much in control of his own medical condition, was quite knowledgeable and was seeing me only to confirm the obvious. Later, I was reminded for the hundredth time that things that appear obvious often are not. He had a pain in the neck.

Now this was no ordinary pain in the neck. It had been so troublesome that at times he could not practice. He had consulted famous rheumatologists, neurologists and finally a neurosurgeon. The first two did not commit but the neurosurgeon applied his talents. Degenerative joint disease with foraminal encroachment of the cervical roots was the diagnosis. Overgrowth of bone was biting at the nerves and giving him pain - so he was told. He had surgery and after six weeks of convalescence he was much improved and he returned to his busy office practice. Now, however, six months later the pain had returned and didn't I think that a simple injection of steroids into the "trigger point" was indicated?

The examination was not very remarkable. There was some rust on his iron. He was after all well into his sixties, had worked hard and a few creaks and squeaks were in order. I could find no evidence of serious disease.

"Sure, a little cortisone here where it's most painful won't hurt you and might give you some relief." He seemed pleased that I would take him seriously and that I would concur with his own planned treatment. I guess I affirmed him and he needed that.

He called the next day to share his pleasure that indeed he was better. It wasn't too long, however, until he was back. Many visits ensued, each with more conversation and less therapy. Over the course of time, I learned much more about my medical colleague. He always regarded me as a colleague not as his doctor. He grew fond of me in a fatherly way and invited my wife and me to visit him at his home.

He was the first doctor in his little rural town having set up shop just after World War II. Like many of his day, his office and home were one. A large pretty frame house on the main street with the office entrance on the side. There was an astonishing array of lovely antiques, majalica, stoneware, ancient firearms and bric-a-brac. As he led us on a well rehearsed tour he explained that most of the pieces had been payments in kind for services he had rendered to patients. He had been dearly loved. Yet there was a bitterness in his monologue rather than fond memories of good deeds.

It is a pattern that I have come to recognize. A pattern of chipped enthusiasm, confused needs and wants, and foggy notions of identity. When a new physician starts practice alone, especially as a family practitioner, there appears no limit to what he or she can do. Show them that you care, that you are available. Go the extra length and bestow on them the gifts you possess. He had clearly been like this when he started. He recounted wonderful stories of bad weather house calls, surgery just in time, difficult deliveries, comfortable deaths, and humorous anecdotes about the farm families he attended. He delivered babies at home, took out tonsils in his office, ran office hours well into the evening every night, never took a vacation, and practiced his trade at church and in the barber chair. There were both smiles and sadness as he told these stories. His sense of personal worth was wrapped in the needs of others. Nothing paid more sweetly than the "Doc, you gotta come!" The rule was to never say no. After all, if you don't do it who will, and someone might die.

So, he never said no. His office was jammed. Appointments that used to be twenty minutes dwindled to five or less. Pills from the barrel were dispensed with less care. He had no time to keep up with the literature. "People need me." He would not press for payments so the payments in kind began - first food stuffs and later more substantial gifts.

As time wore on, so did he. The need he unconsciously curried began to wall him in and become his prison. His jailers, previously friends, never let up. Always calling, always nagging, never understanding that he was tired. "Always thinking of themselves, never considering me" was the last thought before sleep at night. By now the rule, DON'T SAY NO, was a stone tablet around his neck. Money and materia became the solace for these continual demands. If they were to fillet his flesh, then by God it was going to cost. He accumulated wealth, and bile.

It wasn't evil. It was sad. I slowly realized that what he really wanted from me was a way out. He wanted to quit practice but couldn't bring himself to do it. How do you break the stone tablet that has defined your life for so long? He would be abandoning people, he would be failing, he would be saying "I made a terrible mistake." But, if his doctor told him he had to quit, well what could he do. It wouldn't be his fault and everyone would understand that.

"You know, I think you really should hang it up and quit practice," I said casually one day.

"Quit? I couldn't do that. All those people depending on me," he countered somewhat weakly.

"If you keep this up you will really get sick and then what use will you be? Besides, there are more doctors around now and your folks will be well cared for. You've done enough. Why not pack it in and enjoy yourself a bit. You've earned it. I'm telling you this as your friend and as your doctor."

"You really think so. I might get really sick? Let me think about that. I just don't know."

That was on a Friday. On Monday, my phone started to ring. When I came back to my office after morning rounds there were fifteen little yellow phone messages taped to my door. Each one from a new patient wanting an appointment. Perplexed, I called the first one.

"Mrs. Stoltzfus, I have your message. What can I do for you?"

"Well, I need some more of those pills that Doc prescribed."

"I don't understand. Why are you calling me?"

"Cause, that's what the note says to do."

"What note?" I asked getting uneasy.

"Well, there's this note on Doc's door. Says he quit on account of Doctor's orders and if we need anything we should call you at the medical center."

It seemed that he had thought about my suggestion for all of 24 hours. By Saturday he was gone. He and his wife closed shop and went on a three month vacation taking time to put a note on the door of the office.

He passed his stone.

THE RED BRA

BOSTON

Many years ago a terrible fire in Boston consumed the Coconut Grove nightclub and the people in it. The dead and injured were numerous and the local hospitals were hard put to manage. As with many such momentous events there were hearings, editorials, breast beating and proclamations to 'insure this doesn't happen again'. The era of large downtown night clubs came to a close in Boston, the building inspectors got tough and the area hospitals prepared disaster plans.

That disasters will happen is certain and we should certainly try to plan for them but that is easier said than done. Accidents by definition are unexpected so the first variable to work with in planning for them is the time variable. A disaster plan must account for something bad at any time - any time of the day, week, or year.

Even more difficult is to plan to deal with an accident of unknown medical consequences - fire, flood, nuclear explosion, airplane crash, mass poisonings and the like all call for different kinds of preparedness. The Four Horseman had grown to a cavalry.

The plan worked out at the Massachusetts General Hospital was called, appropriately, The Coconut Grove Plan. It began with a cascade of phone calls, which could be triggered from a variety of sources. Then followed a series of actions designed to prepare us to meet any contingency. People arrived, stores were unlocked, drugs and blood made ready, transportations provided, priority listings energized and we would be ready - so we thought.

I saw it used once.

Ice hockey is very popular in Boston. It was Friday night and a well-attended match up involving the Boston Bruins came to a close. A high-spirited young crowd pushed its way to the exits and transportation home. Dozens packed into the double-decked Budliner rail commuter train and hissed off the tracks toward the suburbs. Reaching cruising speed, it had not time to stop for the truck caught on the crossing - a long silver cylinder of fuel oil. I can only imagine the sight.

A dark night with brightly lit train windows as the Budliner split the cylinder at speed followed by an explosion and a rush of super-heated air in, around and through the train - then quiet. Apparently, it was a flash, puff and gone. The wreckage was not great in terms of shredded steel but no matter, the results could not have been worse.

"Coconut Grove!" was called. We knew only that it was an accident on the tracks and that a lot of people were involved. The response was immediate and sure. We got ready. There was secret pleasure in the massing of resources, an excitement to put aside absolutely everything else - this was the highest priority we could have. There was high anticipation as we milled about waiting for the first casualties to arrive. We were hushed and strained to hear the first call of sirens.

They began arriving in twos and fours. First from ambulances and then in cars and pick up trucks. They charged our doors and threw their loads on our litters.

They were all dead.

How could this be? We were ready. We did everything right. We couldn't stop now we had to do something but - they were all dead. The energy to act, to treat, bind, wrap and seal all sputtered and sparked. We scurried about looking for a vent, some not yet corpse that we could work on. One after another, they were all dead.

The bodies were laid out in the long corridor - head to the wall feet to the center, white sheet on each. Two of us trooped the line back and forth snatching off one sheet after another. Surely in the haste we missed one live one. We were ready, damn it, how dare they all be dead. I knelt to one, pulled back the sheet and snapped open a blue oxford button down shirt to listen with my stethoscope. Her young face was black to the collar line with soot. It was as if fine black powder had been applied with care. There was no blood and no singed hair or skin. She had died from inhaling superheated air. The soot line stopped sharply at the collar of the blue shirt. Under the oxford, her skin was creamy white and her young breasts were cupped with a beautiful red bra. There was not a sound.

I don't remember how many died. I will always remember the blackened face, blue oxford, white skin and red bra.

THE STROKE

HERSHEY

"**D**oc, Sara's had a stroke!"

This is the one diagnosis about which non medical people are rarely wrong. They may never have seen one before but the recognition is immediate, almost primitive. Even children seem to know the event.

"What's happened, Sam?" I asked, seeing my evening plans disappear.

"Well, she wasn't feeling too well today. She laid down to take a nap and when she went to get up she fell down and now she can't move her left side," Sam said with a quiver of fear in his voice.

"Ok, Sam, take it easy. I'll call the ambulance and have them bring her into the emergency room. You follow along in your car. I'll meet you there."

"I don't know if I can Doc," now clearly panicked.

It's alright, Sam, the ambulance crew will help you lift her and get her here."

"No, that's not it, Doc. Sara says she's fine.
There's nothing wrong, she says, but Doc she can't move her arm or leg on the left. She's acting real funny about it."

"Sam, listen. It sounds like she's had a special kind of stroke. The kind where she can't tell that anything is wrong. Just get her in her anyway that you can and we'll sort things out."

I called the ambulance office and explained that they would be picking up an unwilling patient. There are often patients who think there is something wrong when there isn't but not too often when there is something wrong and they don't believe it. Waiting in the emergency room, I was reminded of William Carlos Williams short story of the use of force. I could imagine Sam and the ambulance crew horsing Sara onto a litter, strapping her down, grunting down the stairs out into the cold night, bumping into the back of the van and shrieking to the emergency room. Hardly a paradigm of respecting patient autonomy. Somehow, "It's for your own good," seemed weak. In this case, it was probably good for Sam more than for Sara. We aren't very good at fixing broken brains.

They arrived with flourishes and flaps - all the practiced moves of professional emergency workers. Spirited out of the van, quickly down the corridor, double quick lift from their litter to the emergency room stretcher and then a sudden pause. Everyone, Sam included, standing around Sara as if to say, "Okay, we did everything right. Now it's your turn Doc."

Alright, I thought, take control. Use your force. "Put a line in her left arm, get some oxygen running and get me a cardiogram and some blood for the lab," I ordered, more to give some continuing sense of action than because it was all immediately necessary.

"Sam, go out to the front desk and check in. I'll be out to talk to you after I've had a chance to examine Sara." Everyone was glad for something to do except me.

"Hi, Sara. It's Doctor Burnside. Do you recognize me?"

"Of course I do! I don't understand what's going on. Sam just went crazy running around, calling you then forcing me to come here. I'm fine. What's going on?"

"It's alright Sara. Sam got worried about you. He thinks that you have had a stroke. What do you think?"

"Nonsense, Doctor, I'm fine as you can see but I'm getting damn mad about all this."

"Did you fall, Sara?"

"Fall? Uh...well, I guess I did. Must've tripped on the carpet or something but that's no reason for all of this!"

Sara was vacuous and not nearly as quick and bright as I recalled from previous office visits. She was disheveled and frazzled even more than the events would have called for and certainly more than Sara would normally have tolerated. She slowly swung her head from side to side and picked angrily at the bed clothes. She was oblivious to the fact that she had a dense complete paralysis of her left side. Her left arm lay askew and twisted at her side.

"Sara, I want you to lift your left arm."

She looked at me as if I hadn't said anything. I walked around her bed to her left side and, to Sara, I disappeared. I stood there a minute and watched. She picked some more at the blanket and looked frequently to her right but never toward me.

"Sara, look at me," I said. She acted startled, swung her head as far as she could to the right trying to locate me. I was at the side that didn't exist. She twisted around to look behind her but never looked left. The examination confirmed the rest. Flaccid left arm and leg, up-going toe on the left, flat optic discs, a complete left visual field cut not because the eye or optic nerve was damaged but because the entire left signal didn't register.

In the parlance, Sara had a non-dominant parietal lobe cerebrovascular accident. One of the most curious of brain defects. Her entire left world suddenly vanished. It disappeared and Sara didn't miss it because all remembrance of the left world went too.

How could there be something wrong with something that didn't exist?

Sara forced me to think about brains - not one of my favorite topics. We don't understand much about the brain treating brain disease is frequently more expectancy than action. Our maps have improved and a really good neurologist joys at defining the geography of a disease later to be confirmed by the pathologist.

We know that trouble like Sara's was either a migrating clot, a thrombus or rupture of a small blood vessel. Now, I can visualize an errant clot dislodged elsewhere, shot downstream, bumping into bifurcations, hesitating briefly, rolling into one or the other branch by chance until finally it is jammed in a pipe of lesser diameter. If by chance that pipe nourished a particular part of the brain, left leaves. I could also visualize an atherosclerotic plaque finally narrow to closure or a thinned arterial wall split after 65 years of pounding.

Our thinking is not much improved over that of Hippocrates who opined that strokes were caused by overheating of blood vessels of the head with resultant attraction of phlegm or a flow of black bile to the head. Nor is our prognosis much improved from Aretaeus' aphorism that, "Should the apoplexy be severe, the patient will die for they cannot survive the greatness of the illness combined with the misery of advanced life."

The very term 'stroke' shows our ignorance. Stroke - as in struck by lightning, a stroke of luck, stroke of violence, stroke of genius. Or - cerebrovascular accident - accident for heaven's sake. What are we saying? If it's the heart we call it an attack but with the brain, it's an accident. Curious.

More curious is the nature of the brain itself. We waffle in our metaphors of the substance between our ears. The switchboard fusebox model held sway for many years. Yes, we could understand complex circuitry, sparks and melted insulation. Then came the chemical soup theorists - special drops of elixir fitting carefully onto special receptors carrying secret coded messages - all in a pudding of grey and white. We put them together and conclude that Sara dropped a hair dryer into the soup - the shock struck her - it was an accident.

Over the next few days, Sam adapted. He was careful to stay on Sara's right side. He dressed her left side and came to think about life with half a wife. Sara remained distressed by all the unnecessary attention but settled into a routine. At least she wasn't afraid. There was no pain, she hadn't lost anything by her reckoning and well, accidents happen.

SHORT TAKES

MISCELLANY

USUAL AND CUSTOMARY

I have become a usual and customary physician. I didn't plan on it and it happened without my paying much attention. Since I get paid the usual and customary fee I must be a usual and customary doctor. Strange, I thought I was better than that. I thought that because of my experience and apparent success (at least as determined by the number of patients who want to see me but whom I must refuse) that I was better than average. I guess not. I thought too, that when I referred my patients to surgeons that I was being careful to select those who were the best for my patients. The ones with the most experience, the best results and the best doctor patient relationships. Then I discovered that they too were just usual and customary. I guess there is no difference in doctors.

At least I know that my lawyer and accountant are not usual and customary. Both are senior skilled members of their professions and they cost more than some others. I'm glad to pay them more than some others in the Yellow Pages because they are very good at what they do.

I'm not yet accustomed to this notion but it may be changing. I now find out that I can be a discount doctor rather than usual and customary. As I understand it, in return for seeing more patients I can charge even less. I think I know how K-Mart runs volume discounting but I'm not sure how I should do this. I guess the choice is to either extend my hours or shorten the visits. I've already noticed that discount doctors tend to stay together. If I see a discount patient, I have to send her to a discount surgeon or consultant.

I wonder where I can put the flashing blue light in my waiting room.

FUTILITY

It was once suggested that the Patent Office should be closed because everything that could be invented had been invented. This idea now comes to medicine.

We really need to stop futile therapy because we are as good as we are ever going to get in curing disease and relieving suffering. What is needed are strict protocols based on current data that tell us when to cease and desist. After all, if survival is unprecedented why challenge the numbers? It costs too much and fits the definition of futility.

I stumbled onto an old journal in which was just such an article. It suggested that patients with greater than a certain percentage body burn should be offered only morphine and comfort since survival had never before been recorded. Strange, I thought, we are now doing much better than those numbers. If we had adopted that notion, of course, the numbers would have remained the same in a self-fulfilling prophecy of futility.

THE DRUG STORE

Have you taken a look around your drug store lately? Of all the potential archaeological sites for scholars two centuries from now, a modern American drug store would provide a curious commentary on our lives.

As with many other small business establishments, drug stores now all look the same. Just as the mortar and pestle and wonderfully scripted prescriptions have left, so have the individual trappings of individual apothecaries. They are now miniature department stores with an emphasis on "personal products and health items." Fortunately, also gone with the quaint trappings is the lair of some of the most notorious quacks of history. Gone is the Coca-Cola with real cocaine and gone is Dr. Southwick's miracle liniment. What has remained is the attempt to respond to the human wishes and desires for the quick fix.

We seem convinced that we are frail, weak, short lived, lacking in adequate appeal and that each of us is marginal in some precious substance that the truly fine people have in surfeit. Strolling the isles of the local pharmacy is to behold a pill, potion, lotion or salve for every available orifice of the body. Just a pop of this, spritz of that or dab of goo and suddenly, without effort, that magic ingredient will restore youth, vitality, lost years or flagging potency. "Multi" this or "mega" that or at least, "newly formulated" guarantees of relief for basic insecurities. We seem convinced that for anything at all awry with us there is something we can put in our mouth to set it right. We need to let others know that all is well especially by the way we smell. The right breath, hair and face odors, and something special for the underarms and crotches. Pheromones of "I'm all right Jack - or Jill." Smell right, must be right. Next aisle, pastel condoms - just next to the rack for school supplies. That's modern marketing.

I got so caught up in my discovery of the familiar that I almost forgot my toothpaste and deodorant.

HOOF BEATS

Getting the diagnosis is the juice of internal medicine. We love to do it and the chase gives its own rewards. As the clues are assembled we often speak of hearing the hoof beats. We all know that when medical students hear the hoof beats they see zebras. A little bit of seasoning and the internist hears hoof beats and sees a horse. When you get really good at it, you will sometimes hear the hoof beats and get out of the way because nature has already made up her mind.

AN "N" OF ONE

This graph appears in every journal. It indicates study subjects who have been given a drug or had a procedure and what happens to them afterwards. There is always one line that bucks and goes the wrong direction. For most who view such a graph, the effect is clearly evident and the wrong way arrow is merely confirmation that the view is of a biological system.

That wrong way patient has a secret that fascinates me. Why is he/she contrary? Which of the patients that I do that procedure to or give that drug to will fly down he scale rather than glide up? I would get more excited by knowing why one behaves this way than by knowing that most do not.

MY FAVORITE SURGEON

HERSHEY

Really serious internists will tell you that one of their prime responsibilities is to put surgeons out of business. This barbaric enterprise of cutting into flesh must come to an end with perhaps the exception of reconstruction and trauma surgery. We dream of the day when coronary artery disease is prevented by pediatricians and where our magic bullets close the need for cancer surgery, gallbladder surgery, hip replacements and the like. We have already made considerable progress in this holy quest. Surgery for ulcer disease must be at least 80% less than fifteen years ago before the discovery of the histamine blockers. Tuberculosis was at one time the training ground for many thoracic surgeons as they resected lungs, wedges of lungs, crushed phrenic nerves and even put Ping-Pong balls in the chest. Cutting for the stone, as it was once called, has yielded to sonic shock waves with no blood. Doesn't a balloon tipped catheter just sound better than bone saws and rib spreaders?

Alas, we have a way to go before we can contain these monsters to the emergency room. Until then, most internists have a favorite surgeon. When, as is still too often the case, we are forced to seek the services of a surgeon for our patients we do so with care - caveat emptor!

Bill DeMuth was my favorite surgeon. I say was, not because he is no longer doing surgery but because our separation of cities puts him out of my reach. I first met him shortly after coming to Hershey out of my residency training. I had been asked to see a fellow physician from a local community who had been discovered to have an abnormal chest film on a routine check up. The physician was so alarmed that he sought the services of an academic health center thinking, as do many, that this was the source of all manna for human ills. Unfortunately it is not and by the simple expedient of "who's available" I saw him in the office.

He made no secret that he was deathly afraid. His father, he told me, had died of cancer of the lung and it was an ugly death. No, he said, he had been feeling quite well with absolutely no symptoms even in retrospect. The check up had been prompted by an application for additional life insurance.

"How much time do I have?" he pleaded.

"Hang on Doctor, I haven't even examined you yet. You're getting ahead of this thing."

The examination was perfectly normal - the chest x-ray he brought along was not. Neither was it so very scary. "Potato nodes" were the first words from my mouth on seeing his x-ray.

"Why doctor, surely the radiologist told you that this looks for all the world to be sarcoidosis," I said.

"Well, yes, he mumbled something about that but I'm sure it must be cancer," was his sharp reply. I was quickly learning more about my patient. Sarcoidosis is an unusual but not rare disease of unknown cause. The pathology is diagnostic and shows lymph nodes, which have become angry about something and grow a multitude of reactive nests with some large multinuclear cells called giant cells. The usual pattern is to involve the lymph nodes of the middle of the chest causing them to plump up and resemble potatoes on a chest x-ray.

Occasionally, the process extends into the lung tissue itself or other organs and under those circumstances cortisone derivatives are usually given with good results. In the absence of this extension, our usual behavior is to watch and wait as the disease regresses and disappears over months to years. What I was learning about my patient was that this benign information was not getting through his personal experience screens. He might be a doctor in another life but this life in the office was solid scared.

His fear was also a bit infectious. Rarely, lymphoma or a few rare diseases can cause this same pattern of swollen lymph nodes in the middle of the chest. I felt the need to contain my certainty that it was sarcoidosis because of his doubt.

"Well, doctor, of course it could be a rare illness even though it has all the hallmarks of sarcoid. How about considering a scalene node biopsy which should give us the answer and we can do it under local anesthesia?"

"No thanks, it'll probably be negative and then you'll have to go farther anyway and we will have wasted time."

"Well, okay then I'll set up a mediastinoscopy so we can biopsy the nodes in your chest directly."

"No, I want a thoracotomy. I don't trust those tubes for mediastinoscopy. You just might biopsy an artery then I'm in for it. Besides, if its cancer I want the surgeon to see if he can resect it."

It is not unusual for patients to ask you to do a bit less than is required to diagnose or treat and to want to avoid the surgeon's blade but it is distinctly unusual for a patient to ask for more of an assault than is needed. For the gain of time and quick certainty he was asking to be put at substantially more risk.

His reasoning was shot to hell. A scalene node biopsy would almost certainly be positive and it only involves a small incision in the side of the neck. A mediastinoscopy is a bit more adventurous requiring us to insert a viewing tube under the breastbone at the neck, angle it downward until the nodes come into view and take a small bite biopsy. He wanted a thoracotomy. He was convinced that this was cancer and had the unrealistic notion that maybe it could be resected in spite of the fact that it was on both sides of the chest. We reviewed all this but he remained steadfast. He wanted a thoracotomy and he wanted it soon - like tomorrow. I promised to talk with the surgeons and call him later in the day.

Since I didn't know many of the surgeons yet, I asked one of my medicine colleagues for a recommendation.

"If you had to have your chest cracked, who would you have as your surgeon?"

"Bill DeMuth," was the reply without any hesitation.

I found him in the surgery clinic between patients. He was about five ten; perhaps fifty years old, hair a little thin and he greeted me with the most delightful lopsided smile that I took to him immediately. I quickly summarized the findings and complaints and request and showed him the films. I was a bit embarrassed to be making an unusual request especially one, which indicated that I had been unable to steer a patient to the correct path. If he felt that way, he never showed it. He was all accommodation.

"Sure, he said, we can take care of that. How about day after tomorrow."

No arguments, no hemming and hawing, no delays to let me know I was imposing and the supplicant. Arrangements were made, preliminaries completed and the patient was admitted in the afternoon with surgery planned for eight the following morning. As a resident in training, I tried as often as possible to stop in the operating room when a patient I had cared for was under the knife. I estimated that it would take an hour and a half for Bill to get to the pathology where I could look in and see it as well. I went to the operating room at about 9:30, changed into those ridiculous scrubs and little booties, put on the shower cap and mask and went into the operating room.

Bill had his back to me and was intent on his work as he leaned over and down on the patient. The patient was obviously on his side with an arm propped over his head as if in a breaststroke. I stepped up on a couple of stools and peered over Bill's shoulder. To my horror, I looked down to see his hands busy at the root of the lung.

There was no lung left! It had been amputated and Bill was busy tying off various cuffs of airways, arteries and veins.

It's amazing how fast the mind can shuffle through cards. I saw the horror on the patient's face when I would have to tell him that he was right and he had lost a lung. I felt the shame of having been so terribly wrong in my diagnosis, cavalier in my attitude and dangerous in my presumptions. Swallowing several times, I got up the courage to let Bill know that I was behind him. I wanted the awful truth from him directly.

"Looks pretty bad Bill," I said.

Without lifting his head, he said "Yea. Full of cancer.
Don't believe we got it all but it's about the only chance he's got."
Then he finished a tie and straightened up turning to see who it was that was behind him.

"Oh, John, its you. You're probably looking for your patient. He's in the recovery room. This is my second case this morning. Your fellow had some juicy nodes and the frozen sections looked like sarcoid."
Oh sweet relief!

I used to believe that speed in the operating room was a kind of drag race between surgeons.
"An hour thirty six minutes skin to skin," one might boast. I now know that speed is essential. Fast surgeons have sure hands. Their patients don't have to go back to the operating room because of

bleeding, they don't suffer consequences of long anesthesia and they seem to mend faster.

Bill taught me other characteristics of good surgeons that I look for. A really good surgeon can refuse to operate deciding that either what is being offered will not suffice or that the risk is too great or perhaps some inner sense warns them off. Good surgeons are not afraid to hurt people.

Now that sounds strange I am sure but lacking restraint in inflicting pain allows them to hurt swiftly and definitively. The total pain is much less than the tentative assaults of those inhibited at the outset. If you find these things in a surgeon stick with him. Never mind if he spills coffee on his tie, makes rounds on his patients at five AM waking them from sleep, has little sense of humor and is argumentative at medical staff meetings. These have little to do with surgical results. In Bill DeMuth's case, however, he had not only the necessary talents but he blessed us with humor, conversation, diplomacy and citizenship. I later learned that before the Medical Center was built that he had been in practice in Carlisle but steadfastly maintained his ties to his alma mater the University of Pennsylvania. He would make the long trek to Philadelphia once a week to pursue research interests and teach young students and residents. This wasn't easy for a young surgeon, raising a family and establishing a practice for it required at least a full day a week with no compensation.

He joined the faculty at the Medical Center because he belonged there. I'm sure he thought a bit about the change from private practice to academic practice but it was such a natural fit it could not be denied. If there were any doubts, they were dispelled by an incident he related over one of the famous DeMuth lunch table monologues which generally sent us all into the afternoons with a smile and chuckle.

Bill's home was a farm and he loved tending to his ground swinging an axe, clearing brush and planting trees.

"It was a hot Sunday afternoon," he told us. "I was way back on the farm digging a hole for a new tree. I was stripped to the waist and sticky with sweat about waist deep in a hole throwing dirt over my shoulder. I saw a pickup bouncing down the dirt track coming toward me. This fella stopped his truck next to my hole, got out of the cab, came over to me and lay down on the grass full length. He opened his shirt, loosened his belt and said, 'Hey Doc. Check me out will ya? I think I got appendicitis."

"That did it. Back to the medical school!"

THE DIARY

DALLAS

A sk ten doctors about their reaction to patients who come to the office with a diary of their medical problems and eleven will groan.

It takes a fair amount of body focus to make someone want to record it on paper. For some, I guess, it fill empty hours. Maybe it's a way of fighting against other signals that suggest he or she is unimportant. If it's on paper it must be true and it must be significant. Rarely is a diary an aid to bad memory. If anything, folks who record symptoms have extraordinary memories. The importance of the information is inversely proportional to the length of the diary.

Harold Yocum kept the most extensive diary of any patient I have ever seen. Harold was a dapper little guy, standing perhaps five feet four. A local retail clerk, he was always impeccably dressed: sharp creases on his suit trousers (always a suit), carefully knotted ties, handkerchief in the breast pocket just so, highly polished wing tips, carefully clipped nails, and sharply parted hair with the long sweep over the bald spot.

Harold was single and I could never get much social history from him - perhaps he didn't have much social history. He had some college education and had worked as a clerk for many years, but he never chatted about personal activities, friends, or hobbies. Efforts to engage him in such conversation made him uncomfortable, so after a few visits, I stopped trying. Indeed, after a few visits there was no opportunity to try. We had to review the diary.

Harold first came in with a nasty bout of bronchitis following a "flu"-like illness. In addition to the bronchitis, he was hypertensive. His diastolic pressure was 115. There was no evidence of end-organ damage, but this was a level that should not be sustained.

"Harold," I said, "we can take care of the bronchitis. Your blood pressure is up. Perhaps we should do some tests and focus on this a bit so that you don't get into trouble with it in the future." An innocuous introduction to the problem, I thought.

His obvious astonishment said otherwise. He looked at me wide-eyed and his mouth slowly dropped open.

"High...high blood pressure?" he stammered. "You mean hypertension - the silent killer!"

Uh oh, I thought, time to backpedal a little.

"Easy, Harold. It's just a single reading of your pressure and you're not feeling well. It could be a flash in the pan. It's a real finding, you could not have had it long because there is no evidence of any damage. Let's check it again next week when your bronchitis is better."

This did little to reassure him. He went out of the office slowly shaking his head, eyes focused on the carpet, consumed by this calamity.

Over subsequent visits, the hypertension was confirmed. A few tests excluded reversible causes. I instituted medical therapy and made the very great mistake of suggesting that he get a home sphygmomanometer to take his own pressure at intervals to monitor his progress. His diary of pressure recordings grew to enormous proportions. He read voraciously about hypertension, not all in the best sources - National Enquirer, Reader's Digest, Herbalist's Manual. He began to include more and more in his diary - time and dose of medication, general feelings, minor aches and pains, food-stuffs consumed, coffee and cola intake. He even developed his own stress scale and described evacuations in great detail - time, quantity and color.

Soon the volume of material was too much for his spiral-bound notebooks and he began to bring in laboriously typed reports. Through it all, his attitude began to change. Early astonishment became resolution and then a certain glee. Harold had a cause - something to which he was absolutely committed, something terribly important - perhaps even a gift to the world.

Harold bought an Apple. Armed with Excell, he transformed typed pages into reams of data. His pressure was really quite easy to control, but at each visit he had to explore the multivariant analysis on his charts and graphs and tease out the importance of barometric pressure, a glass of wine, or support hose.

While he initially looked to me for advice, he soon felt that his database told more than mine. His questions became theories that he would test on me. He sensed, I am sure, my thinning patience with his postulates.

After perhaps 18 months, Harold stopped coming to see me. On his penultimate visit, I got a surprise. No diary this time - a new complaint. He was having painful urination and a discharge. A quick examination and Gram's stain of the discharge showing gram-negative intracellular cocci confirmed that Harold had gonorrhea. He must have felt that this was the final blow to his standing in my eyes as a hypertension savant, and he went off to find a new doctor.

I was glad that Harold had a social history.

CHOICES

HERSHEY

I checked my notes before going in to see her. It had been a year since I had seen her in the office. She was from a small town about 100 miles to the North and had been sent to see me by a kindly doctor I had known for years. He had been, as it turned out, too kindly as was I.

Rheumatoid arthritis was the diagnosis and my notes detailed swelling and deformities carefully graded and indexed. She had "active disease" I had recorded. Recommendations included aspirin, gold, and aggressive physical therapy. I had given her and her husband what I hoped was encouragement - "...doesn't necessarily mean crippling...always something to offer... with proper attention...we're learning more all the time".

I had made another notation; very briefly, of which I was instantly reminded when I walked into the examining room. It was the odor that reminded me. The thick, sweet musty smell of aldehydes, the remnants of last night's (this morning's?) vodka. My last note in the chart "...moderate the use of alcohol".

Looking at her was painful and it made me angry - angry with her and angry with myself. She was sitting on the end of the exam table elbows on knees with her swollen distorted hands cupped up as if waiting for a wafer. Her eyes were down and hooded with tears rolling down her leathery lined face. No shudders or sobs, just a slow steady trickle. Her arms and legs were toothpicks on a brandied pear torso. Her hair was sticky and disheveled and her dress an afterthought mumu.

George, her husband, retired University Professor was sick too. By the looks of him, her disease was contagious or at least he had been splattered by her despair. He wore the requisite clothes for his station - elbow patched sports coat, shirt, tie and penny loafers. But he was as frayed at the edges as were his clothes. He had splotches of stubble missed by a disinterested or distracted morning razor. His gaze, right at me, both cursed and pleaded.

We exchanged pleasantries with no enthusiasm. As I examined her joints, it was clear that she was in great pain and a lot worse than a year ago. No, none of the recommendations had been followed. The aspirin upset her stomach, the gold meant weakly injections and she was in too much pain for physical therapy.

"Can't you just give me something for the pain? Something that'll help me sleep she asked in a gravel voiced whisper.

"I'm sure if she just got some rest everything would be fine", he added.

Stay away from my boil was what he meant.

What I tried to do, and what I did badly, was to point out that she had choices in life. Panic, despair, and self-destruction, I believe, have a common root in the sense that there are no choices, no options. Too often, I guess, the option is so frightening or unthinkable that it is perceived to be no choice at all. Alcoholism gets this way. The choice to change is for many near unimaginable. The fear of doing without and of being away from the supply makes any status quo the only option. I think too, in presenting choices, I am trying to cleanse myself of responsibility - "It's your decision, you decide." We have come so far recently in emphasizing personal decision-making and patient autonomy that we have relieved physicians of much of their responsibility to be beneficent. There really are times, I think, when we should say, "This is what you must do".

I knew what she was going to choose, what she had already chosen before coming to the office. George had made the choice to ride along with her. He needed the suffering, he needed to be needed, he needed cowardice or he needed bravery - I don't know. I had made the choice last year. I chose not to confront what I knew to be the major illness - complicated, frustrating, time consuming, denied - alcoholism.

There was a long period of silence in the room. I suspect we were all reflecting on our bad choices each blaming the other for having forced them - a circle of pointing fingers. We played out the last act with pleadings and admonishments around. Then they went home. Some time later I heard that she had died. Now I have no choice but to remember them.

INTERFERENCE

BOSTON

Metropolitan Friday evenings are filled with people things. Streets, theaters, restaurants and emergency rooms share the exuberance of "no work tomorrow."

The emergency room of the Massachusetts General Hospital was almost always busy but especially so on Friday nights. The local knife and gun club used us as a dressing room and the stubborn coughs, aches and pains finally became too much and demanded attention. Even coronary and cerebral arteries seemed to relish mischief on Friday nights.

During residency training, you spend time in the emergency room each year of your training. With each year of seniority, the task assigned differs until the most senior year when you are assigned the duty of triage officer. You make very quick assessments of patients at the front desk to find the nature of the problem and the degree of urgency and so direct patients, other residents and staff. At the time, it appeared to be a demotion to be moved from the action rooms to traffic duty. Now, I know that to be the most important task in emergency medicine. You have to make the most difficult diagnosis in that role. You have to be able to diagnose "sick". When mistakes are made in emergency medicine, they can be most commonly traced to the failure to diagnose "sick" when a patient is, or to the diagnosis of "sick" when the patient is not.

This particular Friday night was like others - busy. All of the exam rooms were occupied, the waiting room filled with the walking wounded or sick at heart. Everyone was on a short string, barely civil and wary of his or her own priorities. Clerks minded their mentors by securing the right paper work. If the family doesn't speak English, just shout louder. Residents worked the "iron door" policy - don't admit unless absolutely necessary since an admission will only get you grief from the beleaguered team on the ward. X-ray was backed up - why hurry, we're paid by the hour not the piece. There was no degree of urgency, which hadn't been seen before, and too much sense that it really didn't make a whole lot of difference. Not a very humane place. Far from the high drama portrayed on TV.

A pod of five or six patients had just been dealt with when an ambulance driver asked to transfer a waiting patient to one of our litters so they could be on their way. All of the regular ambulance crews knew to do this. Making them return later because the patient was not admitted taught them that an ambulance ride was not diagnostic of "sick". So, they would wait for the triage before scurrying away.

There was a small lump on the litter. A blanket was tucked around the lump and because it was cold, there was a towel around the patient's head. Peeling off the layers, I found an ancient woman. She didn't move. She was curled in a fetal position. Her waxy skin was pulled taught over a tiny boned frame. She had thin silvery hair, a blank stare and a claw hand of an old stroke. Slipping a cold stethoscope under a fleshless breast, I asked what was the matter not expecting a reply. Her good hand slipped out from under her body and grasped my wrist with strength. Her eyes rolled around to fix on mine and in a surprisingly clear voice she said, "Sonny, I've come here to die and I'll brook no interference on your part!"

I remember to this day my sense of astonishment and shame. Dignity slapped my hand. The shape of the body rarely portrays the shape of the mind. Here was the ultimate in patient autonomy.

She was admitted without a specific diagnosis although I was sure she was "sick". She died three days later. We did try to interfere and she had none of it. Since then other patients have announced their impending death to me and I take it very very seriously.

Is it premonition or planning?

THE MIRACLE

HERSHEY

I first met Hazel at church. My experience with women named Hazel was not of a nature to make me gladly anticipate knowing her Some names, for reasons I will never understand, seem to predict personalities. I had been practicing at the medical school for about five years and in a small community that is long enough for folks to have a word of mouth assessment of your competence. Hazel, fond of word of mouth, apparently decided to seek me out but in her own territory. She was a member of the Altar Guild and took the opportunity of approaching me during coffee after church services in the undercroft - what had become my Sunday morning clinic.

"Do you know anything about blood pressure?" she asked.

"I beg your pardon?" I said, somewhat startled by her blunt manner.

"Simple question," she said obviously annoyed

Hazel was about sixty, short, heavy set and dressed 'sensibly' as she was later to define it. She had on a warm cardigan, black granny shoes and glasses on a chain. Her silver hair was (always) pulled to a tight bun on her crown and she assumed (always) her attack posture - ramrod straight, inclined a bit forward, unsmiling face and very direct stare. I had come to learn that simple questions are not always simple. More than once, I had answered a simple question with a direct answer only to find myself in trouble having to follow up with qualifiers and disclaimers about 'your specific case.'

"I see many patients with hypertension," I told Hazel.

"I should like to see you Tuesday at eleven," she said, whisking her pocket calendar from her cardigan, unclasping her pen and sliding on her glasses. She was about to whirl about and leave when I stammered that perhaps Tuesday would work but I would have to check my calendar to be sure. "Very well," she said. She stood there and looked at me her calendar in hand and pen poised. I realized that she expected me to produce my calendar and we could get on with it. She gave me an 'I gottcha' grin when I said that I did not carry my appointment book to church or out of the office. She sighed audibly and instructed me to have my "girl" call her Monday before ten with an appointment. "Any later and I shall be on errands."

Bun, glasses and calendar appeared in the office later the next week. I was perhaps ten minute late seeing her. "Running a bit behind are we?" was her greeting. "Of course it must be difficult keeping on top of everything with such a small office" with the 'gottcha' smirk again. Hazel was short on love and trust. She had seen many doctors in the area for her hypertension. All were dismissed with similar castigations - just not capable but always with a disclaimer allowing for an explanation other than her own discomfort with them. "... so terribly overworked, don't you know" or "...just getting on in years, I guess" or "...money too important to his wife, so it's said."

I came to understand this later when I learned that she had lost her only child to leukemia at age fourteen. She and her husband, Lester (another name in the aforementioned category) had spent the last twenty years in bitterness and distrust. They were visible in the community in many activities but had no real friends. All of their public works seemed acts of contrition and were performed with astounding conscientiousness and thoroughness but with no obvious joy on their part.

Hazel's hypertension was not difficult to treat but Hazel was. She limited my incursions into her life and well-being. It was fully two years later before she would permit a routine pap smear. She suffered the indignity with expected rejoinders. "Done many of these have you?" And of course, there had to be a problem discovered. Hazel had two large polyps protruding from the os cervix. They were benign by cytology but bled easily and clearly needed surgical attention.

The credentials of the consulting gynecologist were defended, calendars matched for hospitalization, informed consent belabored and she was hospitalized.

I stopped in her room on the morning after admission. She was a "to follow" case on the operating room schedule. This meant she was in line but with no definite call time. "Suppose you have no control over how things are run at your hospital, do you?" was her greeting. "I have a miserable pain in my back," she continued. "Your mattresses are just too soft, but I guess you've never slept on them. I don't know if I shall be able to tolerate this." Murphy visited. I should have expected his law to apply here. The operating room ran late and the last case was the one just before Hazel. The next morning she was gone. The gynecologist was apologetic. He explained that she signed herself out of the hospital complaining that her back hurt too much from the mattress and that we would have to deal with the problem some other way.

My self righteous summary was that Hazel was just frightened of the loss of control that came from hospitalization and the particular loss of control that comes with general anesthesia. She had therefore seized on any apparently acceptable reason to dismiss us and leave the hospital. I was wrong. Her back really did hurt.

About three weeks later, I got a call from the emergency room. A resident explained that Hazel was there and that he thought she had a cord compression. "Cord compression?" I was incredulous but the examination confirmed the diagnosis. Hazel was paralyzed from the waist down and had no sensation below her navel. The pain she had complained about persisted after she left the hospital. She had noticed some gradual weakness and suddenly collapsed at home and was unable to move her legs.

For the second time in her life, Hazel was swept along by events. A compression of the spinal cord is a medical emergency and there was no time for her calendars or qualifiers. Myelograms, the introduction of radio- opaque dyes into the spinal canal, confirmed a complete spinal cord block between the eight and twelfth thoracic vertebrae. Later that day, Hazel was in the operating room where the neurosurgeons decompressed her spinal cord. There was a mass curled around the cord squeezing it in the narrow confines of the boney canal. The pathologists diagnosed the mass as a mucinous secreting adenocarcinoma. Such a tumor never originates from the spinal cord or adjacent tissues. This meant that the primary cancer was somewhere else and that this lesion was a metastasis. The most common primary site of such a cancer is in the gut, but where? There had been no inkling that Hazel was hiding a cancer. She had lost no weight, had no change in stools, no abnormal laboratory tests and no localizing symptoms.

Hazel recovered almost completely from the surgery. Motor and sensory function returned and she was able to walk without assistance.

She wasn't happy. She wasn't grateful. "I told you I had back pain!"

We did the obligatory search. Barium in every orifice, CAT scans, lab studies, removed the uterine polyps, probed and prodded - all negative. "Can't find it, eh? Well I guess we all have our limits."

We decided to watch and wait. We didn't really decide, there was nothing else to do.

A year past with no change in anything. I went to the pathologist and we reviewed the tissue removed at surgery. There was no doubt about the diagnosis - mucinous secreting adenocarcinoma, definitely metastatic.

It has now been twelve years. Hazel and Lester continue their self appointed rounds in the church and community. I don't know if she has cancer or not. I suspect not. I rather believe that a miracle visited Hazel. I have seen three or four miracles in my practice and I think about Hazel's miracle a lot.

Some would argue that the spontaneous remission of cancer is not miraculous only not understood. Perhaps so. The miracle to me is more that this special event should have happened to Hazel - and to me. We think of miracles as divine events and by extension assume that they represent God's grace. Aren't they supposed to happen to the innocent or the holy? Hazel and I qualify on neither account - Hazel was mean and I was delinquent. Perhaps it is miraculous punishment. Hazel lives on in a spiteful life and I am constantly reminded of my failings by her presence in church and in my office. If I finally figure it out, it will still be a miracle.

DENIAL ABC'S

BOSTON

Alcoholism

No more then a couple.
Often not at all. Any time-
Any time I can quit.
Dr., about these headaches.

Breast Cancer

I just noticed it last week.
What do you think it is Doctor?
Certainly not serious do you think?
My that's a pretty tie you have on.

Child Abuse

Just the most active child!
Tumbles and falls, Lordy!
How long with the cast doctor?
Need to run on now, three more at home.

WHO'S THE PATIENT?

HERSHEY

I sometimes get confused about my role in medicine. This confusion especially comes when it is not exactly clear about what is the right thing to do. Not right in the sense of right medicine but right in terms of other actions attendant to medicine. I know that in all respects I should do the best for the patient and keep confidential that which passes between us. But, I am also reminded that I practice by license from the State and that the State financed a large part of my education. In exchange for that privilege, the State expects me to act in the public interest. Others sometimes have expectations on us and trouble comes when what the State or these others want is not in the patient's best interest. Last week was a big week for confusion. Let me tell you of three patients.

Eric Claybell, a twenty-three year old rambunctious underachiever floated along the Pennsylvania turnpike on the vapors of Old Granddad and Iron City beer and whatever else he was provided by the myriad of quick bar friends he casually engaged. Oddly, he thought, he didn't feel too well as he pulled off at the rest stop to empty one tank and fill the other. Copious vomiting followed a wave of nausea in the men's room. This was not an unusual event for Eric except that this time the liquid discharge was more blood than anything else. Although drunk and carefree, Eric was not stupid. He opined that this could be trouble and weaved his way to our emergency room.

It was soon clear why Eric rarely bought his own drinks. Even in his current state, intoxicated and splattered with bloody emesis, he was immediately likeable. He was toe headed, had a toothy smile and innocent gaze and soon had the emergency room staff warming to him and sharing light banter. The nurses, who had seen it all and done it all, were tender to him as they urged a soft rubber tube into his stomach to begin aspiration and an ice water lavage. Their affection went with him when he was sent to the floor.

His alcoholic gastritis cleared rapidly and he had all the time he needed to garner the same attention from the interns and floor staff as he had done so quickly in the emergency room. His room soon became the preferred break spot instead of the staff lounge or coffee shop. Outrageous humor and seeming acceptance of absolutely everything caused his callers to reveal instantly their most private musings. He would greet such disclosures with no serious wisdom but mostly with an energetic nod and smile. "Hey, that's okay." Cigarettes and candy gifts appeared all over the room.

Twenty-four hours later he had rum fit. A grand mal seizure so called because of its association with alcohol withdrawal. We were surprised since he had shown no other signs of withdrawal and he had given no history of having had seizures before. The violent thrashings and bow string tension of arms and legs released quickly to a deep sleep. When he woke he was groggy but no worse for wear.

"Oh, yea," with a great grin, "forgot to tell you that that happened twice before after saucing a lot. Guess I forgot."

The usual studies confirmed that he did not have a seizure focus and there was no structural abnormality of his brain. No doubt that this was a simple alcohol withdrawal seizure. It would not recur unless he drank again and it did not require medication.

We convinced Eric to go to a rehabilitation unit for the next month. His wealthy father thought that was a great idea and surprisingly, Eric concurred.
"Hey, a new gig."

Perhaps the time was right, perhaps he met a special counselor, perhaps something penetrated his bon amie with serious intent, I'm not sure. Eric became a recovering alcoholic. He stayed on at the rehabilitation facility as a maintenance worker rather than return to his native New Jersey. Attendance at Alcoholics Anonymous provided his daily mass. The energies he previously used to gain favor and friends were diverted to helping other alcoholics out of despair. He was very good at it.

Eric visited my office for follow-ups and friendly talk. Before I relate the vexations of a particular visit, let me tell you the other two stories.

Janet Boschwitz at age twenty-six knew almost everything there was to know about systemic lupus erythematosis. This peculiar disease stalks women, usually bright women and sometimes querulous and contentious women. As a group, patients with lupus strive more than any other diseased cohort to form groups and understand their disease. They write newsletters, congressmen, and articles for Ladies Home Journal and diaries for their doctors. Confronted with an illness of variable and sometimes fatal consequences, an illness with no known cause, and an illness poorly treated, one might understand their impatience, frustration and inclination to be wary of doctors.

A sunburn at age seventeen introduced Janet to her disease in waiting. She exploded in a diffuse body rash, high fevers and joint and muscle pain. Over the years, she had episodes of pleurisy, arthritis, fatigue and one serious episode of pericarditis - an inflammation of the thin membrane around the heart. Fortunately, she had been spared involvement of her brain or kidneys. Still, she had the disease and as far as anyone could predict, would have it for life. Such knowledge tempers your perception of the future. We talked of the future.

"Janet, look. No one has a crystal ball about what this disease is going to do to you. You know you might die early and you might live a long life. There's just no predicting. So why don't you try living your life independent of the idea that you have lupus?"

"I know that," she countered. But I can't seem to act on it. Every time I think about changing jobs, going back to school or getting involved with some one, I keep going over the what ifs."

This self-imposed paralysis of action was the most damaging feature of her illness. For years we discussed the most minor modifications of her life style with the caution of momentous decision-making.

Now, Janet wanted to get married!

Nahum Greene was climbing the corporate ladder. He particularly understood the rules of the very conservative corporation for which he had labored for fifteen years. He was quiet, discreet and extremely competent. Nahum was clearly star crossed and destined to make it big. Part of his success was his enthusiasm for all kinds of work. He contributed talent and time not only to the corporation but also to the community in many different ways. It was also clear that he did it not because it would help his career, which it clearly did, but because it gave him real pleasure.

The corporation that Nahum worked for attributed its success to tradition. Change came slowly or not at all. There had to be compelling reasons to discard any operating practice for something new. Quills gave way to mainframes not with enthusiasm for technology but because returns justified costs. Corporate values were corporate rules. You honored contracts at all costs - including marriage contracts. A divorce would break the rung on your ladder. Positions were filled from within. There were no national searches and no headhunters; only the crucible of scrutiny from within would vet you. Nahum understood all this without being told. He was now being considered for a position in the inner sanctum. This was astonishing since Nahum was also a Jew in a Wasp nest and this was not at all traditional.

Nahum and I had a secret. Corporations hate secrets, at least secrets that aren't theirs. Our doctor patient relationship over the years had grown to a friendship. We each knew we could call on the other. We didn't do it often but we were both pleased in the knowledge. I had attended to his annual physicals, immunizations for foreign travel, occasional flu bugs and tennis elbow. Nahum whispered his secret to me through the tubes of my stethoscope when I did his first physical examination. Nahum's heart whistled with a murmur of aortic stenosis. It was probably congenital in origin and tests had shown only minor resistance to flow from his left ventricle to his aorta. There were no symptoms and no outward signs of this secret.

Aortic stenosis can be nasty. The first symptoms are chest pain and faints with exertion. As the nozzle gets tighter, the pressure in the pump rises to very high levels until the pump fails and the stream becomes a trickle unable to sustain life. Eventually, Nahum would follow this progression unless treated. Surgical replacement of the aortic valve prevents death but it is not an innocuous procedure. Even running the gauntlet of gas, knife and blood transfusions, patients with such new valves take anticoagulants for the rest of their lives and risk bleeding. Still, the major decision in front of Nahum and me was not what to do but when to do it. It was a surety to happen at an unsure time - not now but sometime. How long could we suck on the lifesaver before biting down? Next to secrets, corporations hate uncertainty.

These three friends of mine converged on my office during a single week to test my friendship and caring. They came in league asking relief from "them." The jousting sticks were made of paper - Eric a driver's license form, Janet a marriage certificate, and Nahum a report for the board. The windmills of "them" were government, public health, and the establishment all demanding the greatest good for the greatest number.

Eric had found a home and a job. He had a small apartment and continued joy in his new found calling which watered his dry self-esteem sponge. He was now being offered a position with a counseling agency. To get there he needed to drive. To drive he needed to have his license re-instated. To get the license, I would have to lie. That little "do not fold, spindle or mutilate" card contained boxes for check marks by a physician. One box for yes and one box for no and one of the questions was "Uncontrolled seizure disorder." Eric didn't know the legalese of this but I did. The Department of Transportation defines this as any seizure within the last twelve months. Eric's seizure was seven months ago.

Janet knew what her form meant.

"Fucking thing! They want a test for syphilis. Doc you gotta fake one for me!"

Hanging on from yesteryear, we require all about to lawfully join in marriage to prove to the world that they are pure and without spirochete. The problem for Janet was lupus. She would show a positive test. Not because she had syphilis but because her confused immune system manufactured a cross reacting antibody, a BFTS or biologically false positive test for syphilis. The opportunity to plead special circumstance doesn't come about until the first automatic sequence is run which is an investigation by the health department. Still, this process generally stirs no waves. It usually means a few additional inquiries and a few more forms but for Janet, the tragedy was time. She was finally conducting her life without weighing everything on the fact that she had lupus. Wisely or not, this included not telling her betrothed. She could not tolerate the notion that the positive test would have to be explained or that her move to freedom now initiated might slow and stumble.

Nahum's board sent a polite request that he be certified of sound body. Please include, it went on, any details that might embarrass his ability to function at a high level of executive competence. Heart disease was not what they wanted to hear. At the top, that ladder is made of balsa wood and heart disease is too heavy. Nahum said nothing. He just handed me the form and looked me in the eye.

Now, in the abstract, these questions unattached to real people are hard enough. You could argue the prime obligation to patients and that failure to honor that contract brings shame to yourself and your profession. The counter arguments are also strong. Society gives you trust in the licensing procedure and you should not abuse that trust. Moral hazard seems to loom on both sides. The legal hazard clearly marks the State's side of the channel. Should Eric, for instance, have a fatal accident while driving with a license that I knowingly falsified, my guilt would be criminal. I certainly could not be in legal trouble by failing to lie but my friends would suffer consequences.

Hence, I was confused and troubled. Who is the patient? The motto of military medicine is "To preserve the fighting strength" which is not bad until it means that those who can go back to the front get treated before those who can't. The professional sport's doctor keeps the athletes running in order to keep the stadium filled and the industrial doctor is asked to keep the workers healthy in order to help the bottom line. We keep running into ourselves.

But this was not in the abstract. During this week it was face-to-face time. These were friends and these are real forms in my hands. Perjury or personal disaster could be a pen stroke away.

What would you do? I can't tell you what I did.

PAIN

MISCELLANY

Pain puzzles me. I know what it is, everyone does. It is a very large part of medicine and the undisputed king of the beasts with no disagreement at all that it must be delt with above all else. If you can't diagnose the disease, if you can't cure it for God's sake make sure that I don't have pain. When told of cancer, I think most people conjure pain before death. It is a very great dread.

I know what it is but I don't know what it is. Be a clutz with a hammer, crack a shin on the coffee table, grasp a hot handle - everyone's done it, everyone grimaces at the thought but it passes. Conjure pain from an incurable disease and the reaction is now different - it is horror. Time has a lot to do with pain.

Pain is linked to the concept of future. My beagle and I are different this way. She has no idea of future. She might hurt minute to minute but I will wonder how long. When do you suppose evolution developed pain? I have to guess that in some forms of life it is a general alert system rather than pain. A kind of noxious noise that promotes action. The ability to do something physical, to move or otherwise react must have something to do with the phylogenetic value of pain. Trees have no nervous system. They can't locomote so why have pain I guess.

We mix intellect with the signal that comes to the brain to register pain. The basic physiology is quite simple. Generate a signal in a particular kind of nerve fiber and it will take the message to the brain of either pain or temperature. The brain registers hot cold or any of the varieties of pain - burning, itching, and knife like, throbbing - and tells where the hurt is. Start the signal anywhere along the nerve that stretches from thumb to brain and the message is "my thumb hurts". Smack the thumb with a ball peen hammer - "my thumb hurts". Squeeze that same nerve in the arm, neck or brain and "my thumb hurts". A nerve knot in the stump of an amputated arm can still carry the same message "my thumb hurts"- the so-called phantom pain.

This simple process gets much more difficult to understand when the brain sautés that signal with the intellect. I can block the pain signal under certain circumstances - hypnosis, heat of battle, or major pre-occupation with something else. I can make it worse with a focus on it or on its meaning. Pain is always worse in the dark at night. The same cavity demands immediate relief now and is somehow better on the way to the dentist. Then too, the same condition in two people stops the world for one and is a minor annoyance to another.

We know too that some part of the body are painless or register only certain injuries as pain. If I stretch the gut it will hurt but if I cut it cleanly it does not hurt. If you break a bone, the bone does not hurt. Only the covering, the periosteum, can send a pain signal. That and the soft tissues around the bone that are disrupted by the fragments and bleeding. Most of the brain is painless - curious.

Deep pain is different from superficial pain. The pain fibers from deep tissues can be selectively destroyed as in diabetes and in some forms of syphilis. When this happens you get an appreciation of the benefit of pain. Patients with diabetic or syphilitic neuropathy, who have lost the sense of pain from deep structures, will destroy joints. It seems that we need the sense of pain from these structures to keep us from repeated injury. When that sensation is lost, minor injuries become major injuries through repeated use. We rest or otherwise protect ourselves when we hurt. When the pain ceases we are healed and go on. Without this feedback we will continue to walk on a damaged foot or knee and compound the damage.

Leprosy likes nerves. The bacterium will invade sensory nerves and destroy them. Fingers, toes, nose tips and ear lobes will fall off - painlessly. So then we have good pain and bad pain. Good pain that warns and protects and bad pain that comes along for the ride.

Pain is universal but cannot be counted. There is no measure of pain. There is no lab test or x-ray that shows it let alone counts it. In this wonderful scientific world of equations and numbers, the best we can do is "It hurts a lot" or "It's worse or better than it was" or "I can't bear it". Pain is an unreliable chameleon. The signal is simple but the message is so complicated.

Treating pain is also cumbersome and confusing. Just as the intellect and the pain signal are mixed for understanding, the signal and level of consciousness are mixed in the treatment. I can completely alleviate pain with general anesthesia. This relatively simple procedure keeps many doctors busy and is always accorded great significance when recounting the success of medicine. It was the end of brandy and bullet biting for amputations and other surgeries. Still it is not used for pain itself rather to keep pain from getting in the way of other good things like getting that diseased gallbladder out.

The next level of pain control comes with narcotics. Here too consciousness and pain trade off. Given enough morphine, I can put you to sleep. A sleep so deep that you will forget to breathe. I can also swing your pendulum from pain to euphoria described as a delicious rush that begs, even demands, repetition.

Why should a powerful weapon against pain extract such a terrible price? It's almost as if there is an inevitable punishment to be paid either by continued pain or the torture of addiction. It's a silly notion I know but it sure suggests that there is some purpose to pain that we thwart to our regret.

We've become a little more demure about this trade off of pain for addiction and I think it's been a good thing. When addiction was linked to social depravity (it still is, but less so than in former decades) we would ask terminally ill patients to suffer pain rather than fall into this pit. Now, at least we can put some of that aside and allow pain control even to the point of altering consciousness, risking addiction and shortening life. Much of the 'dignity of dying' conversation is around the request that we worry less about the duration of life and more about the way in which it ends. So it is now that patients can inject their own morphine on demand. A special delivery device attached to an I.V. will respond to a patient push of the button by giving a small bolus of morphine to a pre-determined limit of dose and time. Just knowing that is enough to dampen a lot of pain. Just knowing that you are in control, you don't have to call a nurse and wait ... and wait.

Curiously we have also become concerned about the pain of death even when we cause death in retribution for crimes. Garroting, guillotining, hanging, shooting, electrocuting and gassing have now given way to lethal injection. This says a lot about our notion of pain and the concept of cruel and unusual punishment. See, pain even gets into politics.

We all know what it is but we can't see it or measure it. We spend a lot of time trying to understand its meaning. The word pain is often linked with the word suffering. I think suffering is a form of pain but not all pain is suffering even though much of our conversation equates the two or at least makes them handmaidens. I once ran a Med-Line search on both pain and suffering. I got hundreds of citations on pain but almost none on suffering. Medicine at least thinks of pain as its purview but not suffering. Suffering is often used as a way of understanding pain. Suffering leads to the idea of redemption. Some promise of better things on the other side of pain -

Enough of this. I've got a headache and I need an aspirin.

THE ANECTDOTE

BOSTON

S cience tends to mathematics. Taking care of sick people is, however, an individual enterprise. Medical science is frequently likelihoods, probabilities, standard deviations and averages. Sometimes the mathematics and the individual don't mesh. What's good for the average may not be good for the individual. I have never had an average patient.

Doctor Stan Perkase is a very scientific guy and he called me on the phone. An anesthesiologist by training, Stan had overall responsibility for the critical care unit. He endeared himself to the administration with his organizational talents. His manual of critical care procedures covered most every eventuality imaginable. His disaster plan had been adopted by many other hospitals. His secretary's word processor sang all day with reports, census graphs, directives and cost reports. He took very seriously the charge to maximize resources and prevent waste. He acted as a one-man steward of Medicare and the Social Security Trust Fund.

"Hey John, the house is getting kind of full. I'm calling to see if we can move your patient, Harbaugh, to the floor," he asked.
"Are all the beds in the ICU full?"

"Well, not yet but it's Friday and there's a high probability we'll get three and a half admissions today," he countered.

"Three and a half admissions?" I asked, pondering half of an admission.

"Well, yes. See, March generally runs a bit heavier and for the last four years, March Friday's usually fill the house. Three and a half to three point seven five admissions per Friday in March."

"Mr. Harbaugh's a pretty sick guy Stan. I'd feel better keeping him right where he is. Give me a call if things really get tight and we can talk about it."

Peter Harbaugh had successfully avoided doctors for most of his fifty eight years. I had never met him prior to his unplanned visit to our emergency room. A large convention center in our town brings many visitors. Peter's turn came with a meeting of insurance underwriters. He felt vaguely unwell for several days prior to his crash. A tightness in the chest, a little wheezing and a dry hacking cough progressed to extreme breathlessness. The panic of near suffocation drove him to summon help from his hotel room and the subsequent cascade of paramedics and ambulance brought him to the emergency room very near death.

In the emergency room, he sat bolt upright on the litter, grasping the side rails tightly with short rapid harsh gasps for air consuming all of his attention. He was blue and seemed both angry and frightened. Blue people provoke a pretty quick response in emergency rooms. Oxygen, arterial blood gases and chest films almost happen automatically.

It was quickly clear that something was desperately wrong with Peter Harbaugh's lungs. It was not cardiac, it was pulmonary. His blood oxygen was critically low and he was not retaining carbon dioxide, so whatever was going on was clearly acute and not something superimposed on chronic lung disease.

Oxygen molecules instead of meeting warm juicy welcoming sheets of alveolar cells were being refused and rebuffed. The initial chest x-ray displayed only a hint of generalized haziness which was not nearly as startling as Peter's condition suggested. Light banter in the x-ray viewing room kept us from musing too seriously about the implications of this illness. We could all predict a long difficult time or a quick dramatic demise.

Desperate diseases are by desperate measures relieved, or not at all, as Shakespeare sort of said. Desperate measures begin with intubation. When you decide to breath for someone it is presumptuous beyond considering which is why we don't consider it very much. We just do it. Breathing is, after all, a rather personal activity. Together with a beating heart, breathing pretty well defines us as alive. For me to do it for you is the ultimate parentalism. We do it easily and without much contemplation other than the obvious that without it you will die.

After the initial shock of being paralyzed and having a large soft tube thrust through his larynx, Peter was relieved. The suffocating pillow had been removed and his air thirst slaked. Millions of biological engines ceased their screaming for lack of fuel and blue became pink. All was well - for the moment. Now, off to the critical care unit.

When in doubt, shoulder the shotgun and let fly. If death seems near anything is worth a try or so we contend. Cultures were taken from sputum, blood, and urine and broad spectrum antibiotics were begun (could be sepsis). Give him large doses of corticosteroids (could be allergic lung). Use some diuretics (don't want wet lungs on top of everything else). Then tinker with the respirator settings. A little PEEP (positive end expiratory pressure) couldn't hurt and maybe a little more rebreathing tube to add just a dollop of carbon dioxide. The diagnosis was not difficult although the precise reason eluded us.

Peter Harbaugh had ARDS - acute respiratory distress syndrome. We call things syndromes to hide ignorance of causes. A syndrome is nothing more than a concatenation of symptoms and signs. It is reassuring only in that syndromes have been seen by someone else. It's not so strange if somebody else has seen the same thing and put a name to it., If a doctor says that you have a syndrome, don't feel better. Be concerned.

Acute respiratory distress syndrome involves the entire lung and is characterized by a massive leak of plasma into the tiny air sacks.

The plasma lines and cements the walls of these air cells and oxygen can't get through. In children, we call it hyaline membrane disease and in adults, ARDS. Infections, allergies, prematurity, toxins can all cause it but seemingly at random. Even oxygen (too much) can cause it. Peter, for whatever reason, had it in spades. Over the next few days his chest films showed a progressive white out. The plasma leak looked like correct-type spilled on the x-rays.

With the respirator, Peter was alert and sharp but without it for even brief times he became breathless and panicked. With the respirator he could, of course, not talk but he could write. He had a beautiful hand. The kind of script shown on commercials or movie letters. The full rich writing of a practiced hand. Morning rounds were questions from us and letters from Peter. He had wit. The food he couldn't have was awful, he wrote. The entourage around the bed looked worse than him, he wrote. The metal urinal was colder'n than a well digger's ass, he wrote. He wrote and joked but he got no better. We reached an uneasy steady state - on the respirator pink, off the respirator blue.

Peter's family appeared. A stout, honest, no-nonsense wife and two sons all grappling with the fact that their number one was tethered to a machine and not getting better yet still hanging in there. Reasonable questions were answered with unreasonable responses. No, we can't do lung transplants. No, nothing new in research. Yes, we have the pulmonary specialists in attendance and no, we don't know how this happened.

Again, all the King's horses and all the King's men gathered. Clustered about they each rendered advice and counsel in their different dialects. "A little azotemia. Pre-renal and aminoglycoside induced," opined the kidney doctors.

"Ejection fraction pretty good and normal end diastolic pressure," from the heart doctors.

"Might want to bronchoscope him and brush for pneumo-cystis," offered the infectious disease doctors.

Nothing happened. One by one the entourage melted away to more pressing or more promising consultations. Our small team of doctors and critical care nurses maintained an uneasy vigilance and became more distressed. Peter was un-der our skin. His banter continued. How could anyone so sick be so bright and alert? The primitive event of dying ought to be accompanied by more primitive acts and gestures - grunts, moans and coma - not conversation. Peter knew how fragile things were. He also knew of our growing worry but he was careful not to press us. Not because he was afraid of confirma-tion of the greatness of his disease but because he didn't want us to suffer more.

Others were not so patient. One day an ugly fluorescent yellow sticker appeared on the chart. A, not so subtle, message from the Utilization Review Team that Peter had now passed the average length of stay for the admission diagnosis and did we need assistance in discharge planning? We felt impotent and the family bordered on the frantic. Then Stan Perkase returned.

"Full house and one in the emergency room," he announced.

"Yes?" I answered, knowing full well what was to come.

"Harbaugh is the most moveable," he said, tapping his fin-ger on his clipboard.

"Come on Stan. He's one of the sickest here and you know it." "That's not the point. Plug him into the algorithm and he doesn't make it," with an impatient edge to his voice.

When I didn't reply to what he believed was obvious, he continued with his lecture.

"Look, a persistent pO2 of less than sixty, more than seventy two hours of an FiO2 of greater than eighty, a similar time interval of PEEP, and a BUN of fifty puts him in the ninety five non-survival category. Now, there's a bed in the intermediate unit and they can care for his respirator needs."

For most patients, going from the intensive care unit to the intermediate unit means a graduation. A step back from the brink with a time focus that shift to days rather than hours or minutes. They can begin to think realistically of home, a niece's wedding, barbecues in the back yard and changing the oil in the car. For Peter and his family it was the hospice. A gathering place of old sad elephants. He accepted the lame, "It will be quieter and more comfortable" with a generous, "Sound's good to me."

Expectancy and action gave way to vigil. The order of the watch was "Don't just do something, stand there." In spite of this, or perhaps because of it, Peter started to get better. A few patches of more normal appearing lung showed on his chest x-rays. His oxygen status crept up and he could tolerate longer periods of breathing on his own without the respirator. Having draped crepe, we were slow to accept these hints of improvement and chance.

There was no way he could make it, we thought. Two more days of improvement and our rounds became more festive. The gentle repartee between us became real and not forced. We were beginning to rejoice. Then, Peter died.

Weeks of eddying back and forth and desperate inching toward health suddenly stopped. A long Pacific roller crashed on Diamond Head. The code blue was over in fifteen minutes. Sudden apnea followed by a cardiac arrest with no response to body blows, hand bagging respirations, searing watt-seconds through the nipples and long needles into the ventricle and it was all over.

Sometime in the days before, Peter had started to grow a long rubber bullet in the deep veins of his leg. It's weight overwhelmed the tenuous hold of the vein walls and it broke free, ricochetted up the cavernous vena cava into his right ventricle. This turbine shot it the last six inches into his main pulmonary artery where it wedged saying "enough of this nonsense."

Peter Harbaugh almost beat the ninety five percent rule. He was almost outside two standard deviations. Five percent live there and statistically if I keep at it I'll find them. I really want to beat Stan Perkase.

PEAKS AND VALLEYS

DALLAS

What do you do if you peak too soon? It seems to happen a lot to entertainers and professional athletes. The former because of sex appeal and the latter because of bones and ligaments. How do you live with the sure knowledge that the best you are ever going to be at the thing most people identify you with is gone and you are only forty?

Today I saw a forty-year-old ex-actress. I remember her well as a heartthrob in my own adolescent breast and other places. A movie star with her own fan club and entourage, starring in films that could only tolerate perfect teeth, selected flesh and no squints.

She married at her peak another performer starting his climb - a musician. His flame grows brighter and he rankles now at carrying along a clinker from a cold furnace. She's fat and depressed and dulls the dinner conversation. For him music is now not a love but an escape. He dropped her off to see me - another doctor for chrissakes- and ran off to an "engagement", a kiss on her cheek because he knew I was watching.

We quickly got to the histrionics, the stage a bit cramped but adequate for the pacing, exclamations, body twisting, "right here" pointing, snorted disclaimers and stage whispers. A strong recital of this doctor and that doctor, this test and that x-ray, this drug and that injection winding to a pinnacle and collapsing with an "I just can go on with this anymore." What could I tell her?

Start over?

ANGOR ANIMI

MISCELANY

JOHN W. BURNSIDE, M.D.

Danger!
A man of sad anger

Damp eye over clenched fist.
Pulling the past through
A needle of contempt

Throat lumps, gall filled bilge,
Pity gilded guilt stalking
The edge of death

Too old to revise and waiting
Is a waste.

Should I kill you?
Or me?

IT HAS BEEN SAID

MISCELANY

Birds, for the

From the index of Nelson's Textbook of Pediatrics written by his daughter

Prediction is very hazardous, especially about the future.
Yogi Berra

Common diseases occur commonly
Anon

When you're up to your ass in alligators, it's hard to remember you're supposed to drain the swamp.
Anon

Desperate diseases are by desperate measures relieved or not at all.

Shakespeare

I am the King
You must do as I say
Or else
I won't be the King

Anon

Quality Assurance Isn't

Me

HOMELESS BEN

DALLAS

T he Dallas Police found Ben shivering and hudled in an alley corner in the downtown district. He was delirious and was brought to the emergency room. I heard his story from the medical resident the following morning on rounds.

"The patient is about 30 years old and was unable to give a history because of delirium. He is apparently homeless and was brought to the emergency room with a fever of 40 degrees centigrade. The physical examination was remarkable for the fever and a skin rash consisting of erythematous lesions of about 1 cm. in diameter some of which were blistered and others crusted. The lesions involved predominantly the trunk, face and proximal extremities. The palms and soles were spared. The neurological examination showed no focal or localizing signs. His white count was elevated, there was mild anemia and otherwise blood studies were normal. The chest film and EKG were normal. We did a lumbar puncture which was normal. Blood and urine cultures were sent and we started broad spectrum antibiotic cultures. This morning his temperature is only slightly elevated and he is more responsive."

It was the usual succinct and pithy summary I had come to expect from this resident but it was delivered with a tone of disdain. I was getting used to that from him as well. He was well tempered in a sad sense. Parkland no longer held any surprises for him, he had seen all manner of people plights and disease. You could catch him from time to time daydreaming and I guess it was about the private practice opportunities and the relief from the frustrations and fatigue of the county hospital that was on his mind.

"O.K., let's go see him", I said.

Ben was in a fetal position with his back to the door when we walked in the room. He rolled over when he heard us. He had bright red hair and a full red beard both discheveled and dirty. The room had a musty odor. The visible parts of his skin showed the sores with enough clarity to make the diagnosis obvious. Ben had chicken pox - severe chicken pox.

"Hello, Ben. My name is Dr Burnside"

"Ell-uh-whoa."
"I beg your pardon?"
"EL-UH-WOA"

Ben had a speech impediment, apparently unnoticed in his delirious state. His face grimaced with the effort, sound started in his throat and was then forced out through his nose. Once you tuned in he was not difficult to follow except for a tendency to help him by finishing sentences for him which he didn't like at all.

We were in a horseshoe around his bed with the resident on one side, I on the other and the other students and residents in between. Ben was facing me and responding to my questions. The senior resident was off in space, arms folded across his chest and his field of vision about where the wall met the ceiling. Suddenly Ben snapped his head toward the resident and shouted at him. "Don't stand like that. It's too authoritative!"

Now that was a showstopper. No one knew quite what had happened. Before anyone could respond, Ben went on to say, "That's the way the police behave!"

This was the voice of experience. More importantly, we all noted that our surprise was that the combination of homelessness and a speech impediment led us to conclude that Ben was probably also not very bright - a conclusion in error. During his stay, Ben was to continually surprise us with his observations and perceptions of the world from the point of view of a homeless man.

Homelessness has been in the news a great deal. Simple thinkers on the one hand state that all homeless are downtrodden, mistreated and oppressed and that given adequate resources all would choose to live differently. Simple thinkers on the other hand contend that no one need be homeless and that if they are without shelter it is because of the exercise of their own free will. I decided to ask Ben about it.

"Ben, how long have you been on your own?"

"Long time. Left home when I was about fourteen", he replied.

"How long have you been in Dallas?"

"About a year. I was in Mexico for a couple of year before coming here."

"How did you fall on such hard times?", I asked.

"What hard times, I'm alright. People leave me alone and I get along OK. Jesus keeps me out of trouble", was his reply. "How did you get along in Mexico? Do you speak Spanish?" "Can't speak Spanish - Can't speak English as you've noticed", he laughed.

"It was easy, though. I just drew pictures and held them up and showed them what I needed."

He mimed holding a piece of paper beside his head with one hand and either putting food into his mouth or beside a tilted head with the other hand signifying food or sleep.

"Sometimes they would give me money for my pictures. I could get a large poster board for about fifty cents and sometimes get good money for it when I finished."

"Ben, if you had your choice, where would you live?", I asked. "Probably Florida. I have some friends who were headed that way and I would like to find them."

"You mean they live there?"

"No, they're just there. They move around like me", he said.

I told my teenage son about Ben one night and he suggested we get him some drawing materials. We got a thick pack of heavy bond, a six-pack of colored Marks-a-Lot pens and a brown manilla folder with the string ties that lawyers and draftsmen like to use.

Ben was delighted, screwing up his face in a big grimmace making his speech even more difficult to understand. He immediately proceded to make his drawing. Drawing because he only did one - the same one over and over. Soon, everyone on the unit had a drawing by Ben. It was a large flower of yellow petals and green leaves over which he wrote in script "Thank you Jesus for Loving Me - Amen".

"What's wrong with that?"

This was the coin of Ben's realm. It moved him wherever he wanted to go and got him food and money on the way. It was also what Ben most wanted people to "hear" from him.

As Ben approached the dry stage of his skin lesions we asked Social Service to see if we could find him a shelter for his final convalescence. We found instead a very terse note in the chart from the social worker recommending psychiatric intervention. There was the hint that Ben had been rude and a reference made to his "delusional state".

"Ben, what happened between you and the social worker?

"She wanted me to go to the Salvation Army Shelter", he said.
"They talk dirty there and they make m e do things I don't want to do".

Time passed slowly for Ben. He was confined to his room since his chickenpox but contagious. We put a few dollars in his obvious bedside jar so he could rent a T.V. but he didn't watch it much. He wasn't very sick by the third day but we also couldn't discharge him. to the street.

Ben finally got to leave the hospital. I asked him where he was headed and he showed me his bedside jar.

"Florida", he said. "I've got Florida in the jar. Sixty eight dollars here will buy me a bus ticket to Florida. Course, I also have my paper and pens."

I never met anyone like Ben. Maybe there's no homeless person like any other homeless person.

ALZHEIMERS

MISCELLANY

JOHN W. BURNSIDE, M.D.

Lydia Cain's odometer went round
One with zeros turned to zeros unbound
An ancient frame with an ancient sound
Giggles, claps, pouts
Cries on an instant and laughs on a whim
Dribble the food over a liver spotted chin
Dignity is lost – the cry of the kin
Not so bad – a life without sin
She protects the what might have been
"whadyasay, whadyasay, whadyasay?"

Anyway
She sleeps better than she has in years